LUCKY-LUCKY

LUCKY-LUCKY

by Marva Hasselblad

with Dorothy Brandon

Published by
M. EVANS AND COMPANY, INC., *New York*
and distributed in association with
J. B. LIPPINCOTT COMPANY, *Philadelphia and New York*

141497

1

IN FEBRUARY OF 1962, when American involvement in Vietnam was still very limited, and for reasons having nothing to do with government or politics, I flew to Saigon en route to the coastal city of Nhatrang. At the Saigon airport I boarded a twin-engine DC-3. It was a relic that seemed to fly by faith alone. But since a similar faith was propelling me on that day, I never doubted for a moment that we would complete our journey.

Squeezed into a seat scaled to the Oriental physique, in a cabin stripped down to accommodate as much cargo as possible, I was finally approaching my goal. I had dreamed of and planned for this all my life. It was a goal that would hardly seem romantic to most American girls, I suppose, but for me there was no greater romance, or joy for that matter, than to be sitting in this tiny seat, in this battered and cluttered aircraft that was taking me to a place I had never seen; to people about whom I knew very little.

Out of Saigon, the noisy plane flew above jungle flatlands, then headed north along the coast. A lovely young mother hushed her crying child. Vietnamese businessmen and military personnel were engrossed in documents and quiet conversation. And I scanned the jungles behind the coast, hoping for a glimpse of anything that might give me a clue to the adventures and tasks that lay ahead.

My excitement was so great that I was hardly aware of the nervousness that accompanied it. This was my first overseas assignment as a nurse. I had contracted to serve three years at the Chan-Y-Vien, a hospital in Nhatrang, Khanh-Hoa Province, South Vietnam. The hospital had been built in 1961 with funds provided jointly by the Mennonite Central Committee of the United States and the National Protestant Church Council of South Vietnam. Supervising the hospital's entire day-to-day routine would be my responsibility. At twenty-five I thought I was mature enough to handle work that normally, back in the States, would be assigned to a woman much older than I, with years of practical experience behind her. I had been anxious to leave, confident that I could handle whatever would come up. But suddenly, on this last leg of my long trip, I felt very young, very inexperienced, and very much alone.

When I said farewell to my family at Idlewild back in New York City, my mother, who over the years has been separated many times from her children, seemed her usual calm and collected self. My father could not be present—he had, in fact, preceded me to Asia on a survey trip for the American Leprosy Missions. My sister Wyva and brother Carl were at the airport with Mother, both slightly envious that I was traveling over the Pacific. They had been born and, like me, raised in India. Our father, a Baptist missionary doctor, had been in charge of a hospital in the province of Assam. The same stubborn determination and dedication that had led him to practice medicine in India was now sending me to a nursing career in Vietnam. And, more important, it was his example as a physician working under the most trying and primitive conditions that had inspired me to study nursing, and later to apply for a position in a voluntary hospital. Although none of us knew what I would find in South Vietnam, our memories of a happy life in rural India gave promise of good things awaiting my return to Asia. We joked and laughed as we said goodbye—none of us would have dared to cry—and I emplaned for the long journey. The West Coast, Hawaii, Tokyo, Hong Kong, and Saigon were soon behind me. At last, only one more airport lay between me and the Chan-Y-Vien of Nhatrang.

Sitting next to me was Rudolph Lichti, my escort from Saigon. He was director in South Vietnam for the Mennonite Central Committee. The M.C.C. had been set up, decades ago, by Americans of Russian descent as a relief organization to send supplies to their relatives during the revolution. After that emergency the M.C.C. continued in existence, giving aid to refugees and others whom the rushing tide of the twentieth century left in need. Elsewhere in Asia and in Africa it provides medical personnel and drug supplies for local government hospitals, but the Chan-Y-Vien, administered and supported jointly with the National Protestant Church of Vietnam, was a unique M.C.C. project. Mr. Lichti knew better than anyone I had met so far what I would encounter at our hospital. He, like me, had come to a ravaged country with the hope that he could alleviate great and needless suffering. Neither of us was a missionary, although we were both associated with a voluntary organization. Both of us—perhaps he more than I—had left a great deal behind so we could serve where we felt we were most needed.

During the last few minutes of our flight he told me that Nhatrang, blessed with low humidity, had once flourished as a seaside resort for French government officials and wealthy French and Vietnamese businessmen. Although the country had been at war for more than twenty years, Nhatrang, on the surface, seemed unchanged. Most of the 80,000 Vietnamese living in the city pursued life much as they always had. The city was still a resort favored by Saigon members of the diplomatic corps and high-ranking government officials who vacationed in the villas that formerly belonged to the French.

Mr. Lichti said one of the problems to be encountered in Nhatrang and elsewhere in the country was the shortage of Vietnamese doctors and nurses and other trained personnel available for work in non-government hospitals and clinics. Those who weren't working in military hospitals were attached to the provincial hospitals operated by the government, one of which was in Nhatrang. As a result, we at the Chan-Y-Vien had to rely on unskilled Vietnamese workers. In time, thanks to our training, many of those whom we employed at the Chan-Y-Vien would become skilled, but the problem of working with people who had absolutely no experience would continue.

As the plane approached Nhatrang, Mr. Lichti pointed out some of the landmarks below. At first, all I could see were specks of color outlined against the lush, tropical hills on one side and the glistening white beach and bright blue sea on the other.

As we neared the airport, we swung out over the sea and then turned inland. Mr. Lichti pointed out two saffron-yellow buildings roofed with crimson tile just past the beach

8

—the hospital and the house for the staff. As quickly as they appeared they were gone, and we were over the runway. I was in Nhatrang at last.

Minutes later I was standing in the shadow of the plane shaking hands with Eleanora Weaver, the nurse I had come to replace.

The professional staff at the Chan-Y-Vien (the words mean "Charity Clinic") was supposed to consist of a doctor and two nurses, if possible. Each received fifteen dollars a month, plus room and board. The hospital itself received $150 a month for maintenance, drugs, and supplies. The professional staff and its salaries, and the hospital's allotment, were provided by the M.C.C. The co-sponsor of the Chan-Y-Vien, the National Protestant Church Council, provided the native staff and the board of directors, among other things.

I was disappointed that Dr. John B. Dick, chief of the hospital, hadn't come to meet us, but then I realized that the pressure of his duties had kept him away.

Miss Weaver was welcoming me as if I were a long-lost relative. "I can't begin to tell you," she said, "how very glad I am that you're finally here. I've had nightmares during the past few weeks that you wouldn't come, that I'd be stuck here indefinitely." She laughed to imply that she was only joking. But it was apparent that she meant what she said. And I was momentarily disturbed.

Eleanora was in her thirties—a small, slender woman of reticent manner. She was about to terminate three years' duty in South Vietnam, a major portion of which had been spent working with the Rhadde tribespeople in Banmethuot, a town inland from the coast.

The Nhatrang air terminal, a pleasant, vine-covered building, was practically deserted. We waited under a shaded portico while Mr. Lichti stood with the other passengers near the plane until the baggage was removed.

To make conversation I asked Eleanora what the high-collared, long tunics worn by Vietnamese women were called.

"It's an *ao-dai*," she told me, pronouncing the word "ao-yai" and explaining that Vietnamese was a dreadfully complicated language of fine subtle tones. She said she had learned to speak with the tribespeople, whose languages are very different, but during the half year she had been at the Chan-Y-Vien, where only Vietnamese was spoken, she had relied a great deal on an interpreter.

I refrained from telling Eleanora that I was determined to break the language barrier as quickly as possible. Since I had learned to make myself understood in Assamese as a child, I hoped to pick up Vietnamese with equal ease. I was sure it would be only a matter of weeks before I could be speaking simple phrases, and that not many months would pass before I became passably fluent. No matter how difficult Vietnamese was, I knew that, if I were to work with patients effectively, I must be able to communicate with them directly.

Mr. Lichti and my luggage joined us and we went out to the front of the airport where the hospital automobile was parked. "Automobile" was a particularly kind euphemism for that vehicle. It looked like the granddaddy of all jeeps, a broad, high and square Land-Rover which had faded to washed-out gray from apparently a much deeper color.

When the petite Eleanora jumped in behind the wheel, I was more than a little surprised. The Rover simply didn't look like the kind of vehicle a tiny woman could handle. But when she told me, quite matter-of-factly, that she did, indeed, drive it and that I would have to learn to handle it as well, I got my first lesson in the facts of life at the Chan-Y-Vien. Before long I, too, would be handling this ugly automobile like a veteran truck driver.

I hoisted myself with both hands into the cab, banging my head for the first of many times. Mr. Lichti followed with contrasting agility, obviously born of experience. And then I settled back as comfortably as I could to enjoy my first look at Nhatrang.

As we drove from the airport, I saw Vietnamese work gangs and several American overseers along the single runway. Mr. Lichti, who had observed this activity also, answered my unspoken query.

"The runway is being extended to accommodate jet fighters. The American foremen are employed by a stateside construction company under contract to the U.S. Army. It's beginning to look as though the war may get to Nhatrang."

On his last trip—Mr. Lichti came to Nhatrang almost monthly—he had seen local port facilities being enlarged and had heard that an American Army field hospital was to be set up in tents adjacent to the airfield.

We drove out of the airport along a two-lane highway with hedges down the center and turned into the Beach Highway, a beautiful road running the length of the shore. It ended, I was told, at a point that was the site of Francois', a restaurant known throughout Southeast Asia as one of the best places to eat lobster. Later I would often confirm the truth of its reputation. But now we went in the opposite direction. On our right was a bright sandy beach, a blue expanse of ocean, and in the distance some scrub-covered islands. On our left were beautiful villas set in gardens, and beach houses where refreshments were sold, set in their own palm groves. Brilliant bougainvillea clung to the low walls and fences and clustered around porches, a touch of brightness amid the lush greenery. The warm February sun was welcome after the bad weather in Tokyo and Hong Kong, where I had been earlier in the week.

We couldn't see the town from the Beach Highway, but after a while we turned left toward Nhatrang. The bicycle-choked streets and colorful shops provided a sharp sudden contrast. It seemed a clean town—especially by comparison with India, which I now vividly remembered. On the main street there was one tiny shop after another. Shoes, cosmetics, handbags, rain paraphernalia were arranged in front of their respective stalls. Even bicycles were hung, precariously balanced, where they could be seen by prospective buyers. The proprietors, my companions explained, lived either in one room or two behind their shops, which were shuttered at night. In front of the town market were the flower vendors' stalls, and the scene here was even more colorful with gladioli and chrysanthemums in dazzling shades. I was told they had been brought from Dalat, a city located in the hills to the northeast.

Our Land-Rover passed crowded small buses, pony carts and trucks laden with produce and merchandise, and two curious types of vehicles that served as taxis. There were dozens upon dozens of cabs that had been built over Lambrettas—Italian motor scooters. But even more prevalent was a conveyance in which a man sat up high straddling one wheel and peddling vigorously while in front of him a cab, suspended low over a base of two wheels, held his passengers. "These are *xich-los*"—Dr. Lichti pronounced it "seke-lows"—"or tricycle taxis, and a ride from here to the hospital costs twenty-five piasters or about thirty-five cents." They usually held two or three Vietnamese, but sometimes a mother and all her children crowded in.

The Vietnamese are a small people, an old and handsome

12

race, who go slowly and quietly about their business. All the women, young and old, wear trousers—black if they are elderly or belong to the peasant class—and either hip- or ankle-length tunics in a wide range of colors. In contrast, the Western-style dress of the men and children is drab and commonplace.

I commented on the surprisingly efficient management of the heavy traffic by Vietnamese policemen stationed at the intersections. So far, Eleanora said, the bridges and highways leading to Nhatrang had not been damaged by Vietcong dynamite, as was the case in other parts of South Vietnam. The accessibility of the city accounted for its bustling traffic. No one could foresee the future, so everyone lived from one day to the next, expecting that sooner or later the Vietcong would make sorties on nearby provincial roads and bridges.

My heart grew heavy at this intimation of danger to come and my mind filled with questions I had refused to consider until now. I did not fear for my own safety, but wondered how destruction by the Vietcong might affect our work at the hospital.

My thoughts were interrupted as we left the town and approached a narrow unpaved road. I recognized the two brightly colored buildings I had seen from the air.

2

THE CHAN-Y-VIEN. Before me were the two buildings I had seen from the air. On the left, set in a grove of palm trees, was the longer of the two, the hospital, and on the right the bungalow where I would live with the rest of the staff. As we pulled up to the "carport"—a slab of cement over the driveway between the two buildings—I noted the opaque windows at one side of the hospital building that indicated the operating room. While we parked, a man of medium height emerged from the bungalow followed by three small boys.

These were the Dicks, father and three sons. While Mr. Lichti introduced us, I could feel the youngsters, boys of six, four and two, looking at me from all angles. Dr. Dick gave me a quick head-to-toe glance followed by a handclasp and a friendly smile. My own appraising glances at them occompanied the wary small talk and inevitable confusion that attend arrivals anywhere.

And I wondered, as I always wonder when meeting

14

people for the first time, what kind of impression I was making in those first awkward minutes of confrontation.

I am best described as a large girl, although five feet, seven inches is not unusually tall by American standards. My hair is blond, my eyes blue and somehow, regardless of how much effort I make with my appearance, I always manage to look as though I just stepped off the farm—healthy, strong, and slightly windblown. I have the kind of face that a milk advertiser might put on a billboard, but it would never get a second glance from a perfume adman.

I'm also rather shy, which one might think strange, considering the large variety of places I've been to and people I've met. And somehow I often find myself making the most inane remarks—if I'm not totally tongue-tied—when meeting people for the first time.

In this particular situation a set of personal statistics had preceded me to Nhatrang, probably forming an initial impression that my appearance would merely confirm. And as misleading in their painstaking accuracy as these facts were, they undoubtedly laid the cornerstone for my reception that day.

What my dossier reported was that I had spent most of my childhood at a Baptist mission hospital near Jorhat, in the province of Assam, India, where my father was chief medical officer. Most of my elementary school education in India was provided by my mother, aided by correspondence courses from the United States, and later I attended mission high school in Kodaikanal, south of Madras. As for my professional training, I received a bachelor's degree from Ottawa University near Kansas City, and studied nursing at Columbia Presbyterian Medical Center in New York. My training had been completed only two months prior to my arrival in Nhatrang.

Those were the facts. The intangibles—the things there is

never room for on printed questionnaires—I hoped my colleagues would seek out and learn for themselves in time. For now, my nervous smiles and polite small talk would be judged by them as I judged their own.

Mrs. Dick joined her husband and sons and led us out of the blinding glare of the sunlight into the cool darkness of the bungalow we would all share as one family. It was a relief to be out of the midday sun. But it was even more of a relief finally to see the people and the place I had imagined for so many months.

The Dicks were a Canadian couple in their thirties, he quite reserved in manner, she spirited, vibrant, and apparently very content in her role as mother and wife. Not a nurse, Mrs. Dick took no part in the operation of the hospital, and devoted her attention to her children and husband, and to maintaining the building that was home to all of us.

The bungalow itself was a modest version of a suburban-development house in the States. It was of saffron-yellow stucco outside (as were most of the buildings I had seen during the drive from the airport) with a small entrance porch. The front door had a glass panel and was flanked by narrow windows, also fitted with glass. All the other windows in the house had louvered shutters, as is generally the custom in the tropics. The square living room ran through the center to a back door. The living area was on one side and the dining area on the other. Two large windows in the rear framed an area filled with bougainvillea. Two bedrooms and a bath opened off an enclosed hallway on either side of the living room. For some reason all of the interior was painted dreary gunmetal gray.

We chatted first about my trip, then about getting accustomed to the climate, which was not as hot as I had anticipated. All the while I was extremely eager to hear about and see the hospital. I must have forgotten how slow the pace is in the tropics, for I seemed to be the only one impatient to get to work.

My room was also painted gunboat gray, but with windows facing the yard it was brighter than the living room. I took a few minutes to comb my limp hair and wash my dirt-smeared face, and then I joined the Dicks, Eleanora, and Mr. Lichti for lunch.

My first real exposure to Vietnamese foods was embarrassing. I'd never used chopsticks before and the long table, set up boarding-house style with condiments, serving bowls and platters of food ranged down the center, didn't seem to be the place to experiment.

I promptly admitted inexperience with chopsticks. Mrs. Dick came to the rescue with a fork. "We all found—and I'm sure you will too," she smiled, "that Vietnamese food doesn't seem to taste just right with Western implements. Chopsticks definitely make a difference and you'll find them easy to use."

I resolved to learn to eat native food in native style while taking my first taste of the local cuisine with a fork. Everyone pretended to be absorbed in a discussion about drug supplies while, out of the corners of their eyes, they watched to see my reaction to the food. I had expected the various dishes to be hot and spicy, similar to the Indian food which I adore, but surprisingly the meat and vegetables were, although good, quite bland. My face must have betrayed my disappointment, for Dr. Dick promptly offered a condiment bottle.

"Try some of this sauce," he said. "It's *nuoc mam,* and it smells like rotten fish, which it is. But it's quite good, and it will pep up the food."

I sprinkled it hesitatingly over my plate, and tasted again.

The smell of the *nuoc mam* (Dr. Dick had pronounced it "nook mom") was simply incredible and I had a hard time getting the fork to my mouth. But since everyone was now watching me, making no pretense at conversation, I at least had to taste it. To my surprise it was delicious. I said so, and everyone was relieved.

I was being treated like a tenderfoot, which I didn't mind in the least, but it made me aware that I had been a little smug in thinking how easily I would fit into things here. I had expected that my previous experience in India would make my adjustment to Vietnam a very simple matter. In fact, I was to find more differences than similarities between the two countries, and it would take some time before I was fully acclimated to the ways here.

I sampled everything on the table. A dish of crisply fried pork in a pungent sauce was particularly good, and so was the crusty French bread that was also served. Fresh papaya, the ambrosia of Asia, completed the meal. And casual conversation, the ambrosia of all civilization, was the perfect after-luncheon sweet.

But was it my imagination that the subject of the hospital had been assiduously avoided? We spoke of many things— from childrearing to the political situation in Vietnam—but not a word about the Chan-Y-Vien. I thought it might be impolite to bring it up, and so contented myself with speculating on what I would find.

Finally, lunch over, Dr. Dick suggested that Eleanora Weaver take me next door and show me around before she held afternoon clinic. I literally almost jumped into my uniform, the fatigue of travel vanishing in an instant. When we left the bungalow it was mid-afternoon, hotter than when I had arrived, but with a refreshing sea breeze stirring the young palms as we approached the hospital. I was surprised that there were no flowering shrubs on the grounds, but Eleanora explained that it was too near the sea for them.

She was not a talkative person and I soon realized that, while she dispatched her duties with professional exactitude, she was so close to the end of her tenure in South Vietnam that she wished to avoid being saddled with additional administrative responsibility and was only too glad to have me take the reins in both the clinic and the ward. This is not said in the spirit of criticism; Eleanora had already done more than her share among the tribespeople. But the final seven months of her three-year tour in South Vietnam burdened with the task of setting up a new hospital had simply worn down her initiative.

"Mimmie, our interpreter, will present you to the odd assortment of staff workers we have been able to attract to the Chan-Y-Vien," said Eleanora as we approached the front verandah of the hospital. I recalled Mr. Lichti's words about the unskilled staff as she continued.

"It is necessary for Mimmie to speak yards of Vietnamese to get a simple idea across. She's a fine girl with infinite patience—a quality I personally now find in short supply."

There were several forlorn and apparently poor Vietnamese peasants—one a very old man—squatting on mats on the front verandah. Eleanora said that they had arrived too late for the morning clinic that ended at noon; they were foot travelers and too far from home to return and then come back again for afternoon clinic. And so they had waited through the noon break period.

I looked into the eyes of a very young woman holding an infant wrapped in rags. The rest—perhaps a dozen men and women of various ages—mumbled what I took to be polite salutations.

We entered the large, bare reception room, furnished only with a desk and a few chairs and lined with medicine cupboards on one side with counters under them for dispensing drugs, and a work area and counter for sterilizing supplies on the other.

"This is where our outpatients are interviewed," Eleanora continued. "They line up on the verandah, as you've already seen."

I asked how many outpatients, on the average, came to daily clinic. She said there were usually between thirty and forty.

Only thirty or forty? I was surprised at the low number. I had expected—what?—double, triple, quadruple that amount? The hospital was still new, but obviously the Vietnamese in Nhatrang had not yet come to accept it. It was the first hospital in the area run by Westerners, and it was quite possible that people were wary of being treated by foreigners. Months later, after I had had occasion to visit the only Vietnamese hospital in Nhatrang, the Province Hospital, I learned still another reason why attendance was low. The treatment they received at their own hospital was, unfortunately, inadequate by Western standards. The death rate there was high by any standards, because the sick traditionally preferred to remain at home, going to a hospital only when they were so ill that they believed there was no other hope for them. Eventually, we at the Chan-Y-Vien would be seeing over two hundred people a day in clinic and the ward census would quadruple. This would be the result of a great deal of patience and effort on our part, abetted by the passage of time.

Three young men and a slender girl wearing the traditional *ao-dai* over full white trousers came into the reception room while Eleanora was showing me the records and explaining clinic procedures. They waited quietly until she finished, and then the young girl was introduced.

This was Mimmie, our interpreter, a girl of delicate features and childlike build. She smiled directly at me. "Happy to meet our new nurse," she said very seriously, in a soft whisper-like voice. And then she introduced the other workers.

They were all young, and they worked for a pittance. They came from in and around Nhatrang and had been trained by Dr. Dick and his nurse to perform routine hospital chores.

Mimmie introduced the oldest of them first. "This is Anh Tin, our sweeper," she said. "He wants to become Doctor's assistant."

I looked at the barefoot young man in front of me. He was dressed all in khaki, as were the other men, but he was more sturdily built than they. I held out my hand and, imitating Mimmie's pronunciation of his name, repeated it. I asked what his responsibilities were, and learned that he swept out the clinic room and verandah before and after each clinic session; that he scrubbed the ward floor twice a day, and brushed out the window sills once a week. In between he helped out in the ward. "I know you must work very hard. I'm pleased to meet you," I said. He smiled and nodded as Mimmie translated my words into his tongue.

"Anh Tin says please thank you," translated Mimmie. Then she introduced the other young men, and I spoke a few words to them too. Only about seventeen years old, they were responsible for taking temperatures, giving injections, keeping the record books in the clinic and giving drugs to both clinic and ward patients. In addition to translating, Mimmie also performed all of these chores.

Eleanora was anxious to complete my tour of inspection before clinic time. "Let's look into the ward now," she said, brushing away a fly that had settled on her arm with a gesture of finality. She led me through a double door, and Mimmie followed us.

The ward was quiet; the only noise came from the buzzing of an abundant number of insects. Of the fourteen beds only five were occupied. Each patient lay on a smooth grass mat placed over the wooden slats of a white metal bed frame. I looked at the patients and, when they noticed that I was observing them, they stared back. Two of the five were young women, one with a newborn infant at her side. Two were men, and the last was a boy so emaciated from malnutrition that he seemed little more than skin and bones. I was surprised to find men and women together in the same ward; Eleanora explained that this was a common practice in Vietnam.

I looked again at the younger of the women. She was just a girl, really. Then I noticed that an even younger girl, hardly more than a tot, was perched on the bed fanning her. I had already been told that members of the patient's family had to provide food and bedside care. I assumed the two girls were sisters—both had beautiful thick black hair and the same large, frightened eyes. They were so small, so precious that I had all to do to keep myself from going over to them.

I asked Eleanora about the sisters and she smiled wryly. "They're mother and daughter," she told me. "Yesterday the mother delivered a dead baby, which was followed by a postpartum hemorrhage. It was her fifth child in as many years and the burden was too much for her. We never expected her to pull through. That little one is her oldest child."

My heart went out to these two until I thought it would break. I asked why such a little child should have to attend her mother and be exposed to illness, tragedy and death in the hospital.

Eleanora nodded her head in a gesture of futility. "We get bedside attendants even younger. The amazing thing is that they're all as responsible as adults.

"From the time a Vietnamese child learns to walk," she continued, "he shares in household chores. These children rarely played or laugh from sheer joy. The nation, the village, the family—they've all been impoverished from so many years of war. And it's more than a matter of money and food. Emotionally, you'll find, they're drained. They've lost their fathers and their husbands and their sons. They've lost their homes and their neighbors and friends. And the worst part of all is that they know the end isn't in sight."

We both were silent for a moment. Suddenly I felt utterly exhausted. The long journey, the trip through the city, the introductions, the visit to the ward, the young mother and child, the job that lay before me—I felt as if my whole being would collapse from fatigue. There were so many things to think of. There was so much to do.

I looked around me again, at this strange ward, two-thirds empty. Why, in a hospital built to serve a city of 80,000 as well as a large rural area, were there only five patients in bed? What could be keeping people away?

We returned to the reception room. Eleanor at once began interviewing clinic patients; Mimmie heard the complaints of the sick and carefully translated the symptoms. As an onlooker, I listened and watched—and blessedly forgot my doubts and fears. The scene before me now brought back my early experience at the mission hospital in India. Memories that I had resolutely put out of my mind during my eight years of study in the States came flooding back.

3

I AWOKE THE next morning with a start. Since no ray of light entered the unfamiliar bedroom, I wondered what had awakened me. Then I became aware of the heavy silence. Not a single sound, not even that of a night bird or night insect, penetrated into the dark, quiet house.

I smiled, realizing that the silence was precisely what had put an end to my sleep. That was one of the strange and wonderful phenomena of Asia. When darkness pales, long before the human eye can perceive the subtle changes in the sky, the night creatures suddenly become quiet. And then, quite gradually, it's dawn.

A new day; I felt marvelous. The strain and fatigue of yesterday were gone, replaced with a wonderful feeling of anticipation. Throwing back the sheet and cotton blanket that had been ample cover against the night air, I felt my way out of bed. As I had expected, I was slightly stiff. It would take a few days to become accustomed to sleeping on the foam rubber mattress that rested on the wooden bedstead.

The house was still quiet and I decided to go down the path to the beach, which I hadn't yet visited, to watch the sunrise. From the end of the path, I could see an enormous rock formation that extended into the ocean a little distance on my right. And on the left was a beautiful cove. The sandy beach extended for about a quarter of a mile between the cove and the rocky promontory. It was like a glimpse into paradise for me, and I knew then that the rocks and the cove would become a haven and a hideaway; a place in which to retreat and think and dream as long as I was at the Chan-Y-Vien.

By the time I reached the edge of the water, the sun was over the horizon. Flamboyant colors blended overhead— piercing blues, wonderful oranges, purples, yellows, and reds—and softly reflected on the sea and sand. I felt the kind of oneness with nature that men and women must have known constantly before civilization intruded into their lives.

In silhouette against the bizarre brilliance of the sunrise I saw the humps of several islands. Then, phantomlike, the sails of boats began to appear. These would belong to fishermen hurrying home after a busy night. I waved to them, but they were too far offshore to see me.

Still excited by the natural beauty that surrounded me, I turned from the sea and followed the road up the hill. I brushed the perspiration from my forehead. The sun was already bright and hot. From the top of the bluff I could see the rivers and the red roofs of the houses in the city. A few cyclists and carts already crossing the bridges were the only moving things in sight.

It was almost six and I hurried back to the bungalow, but nobody had yet begun to stir in the house. I returned quietly to my room to finish unpacking, then took an ice-cold shower and put on my uniform. Suddenly I felt quite famished. In the hope of finding a pot of coffee brewing in the kitchen, I tiptoed out of the rear door, through a roofed breezeway, and into the kitchen house.

Ba-Muoi, the cook, whom I had met only briefly the day before, had already arrived from her home and was at work. She nodded and put a pot of water over one of the butane stove's two burners. As in India, there was a mortar-surfaced table with square wells set in the top that could serve as an additional cooking area. A small portable metal oven was off to one side, ready to be moved where it might be needed for baking or roasting. A sink with running water, cabinets for groceries and the kerosene-fueled refrigerator completed the facilities for food preparation. The kitchen house also contained an extra bedroom and bath, and a storage area for our drug supplies.

The cook went about her business, washing and arranging fruit for the family breakfast and taking down tinned bacon for frying. When the water boiled she brewed a fine cup of powdered coffee. I couldn't have been more pleased—if only because she didn't resent my presence in the kitchen, as did most Indian cooks.

Breakfast with the Dicks and Mr. Lichti at the family dining table was merely routine. Eleanora said she had heard me up before the crack of dawn. I told of having gone to the beach and asked if the cove, which looked so inviting, was safe for swimming.

"I don't swim," she said, "but I go there all the time and see small boys, naked as jaybirds, thrashing around in the surf, so it must be safe."

"But I must tell you," she went on, "Vietnamese women,

26

who are extremely modest and guard their skins from tanning, might be disturbed to see you in a bathing suit and swimming."

I had noted, in fact, a bit to my surprise, that most of the Vietnamese I had seen were quite fair-skinned. And, strangely, the women were almost always more fair than the men, except for the rural people. I realized that lightness of skin was probably something of a status symbol. Since this was the case in most of the rest of the world, I assumed it was not any different here.

I was anxious to get to work, and breakfast seemed to take hours. But finally we were through. Eleanora and I talked over the workday ahead. We decided that it would be best, in the beginning, if I continued to observe how she handled outpatients.

Before morning clinic began we stopped off in the ward. Unlike the day before, there was a happy feeling of activity. Each of the patients was being served and fed by a member of his family, some by a child.

I asked about the food arrangements, wondering how, without a communal kitchen, the patients' meals were prepared. Eleanora told me that each morning whoever was attending the patient would bring the day's food from home. Meals were cooked over charcoal fires out in the open behind the hospital.

She said I would also see food vendors coming to sell such things as French bread, rice, noodles, soups, and meat and vegetable dishes from portable steam wagons. The boiled squash or spinach and everything else was always flavored with *nuoc mam*. Food was dispensed at all hours of the day, with frozen ices much in demand toward late afternoon. But occasionally what the vendors sold was beyond the income of some of our sick.

"I might warn you," she added, "that there's always quite

a smell out by the rear cooking area. Refuse is collected and burned only once a day. This isn't as bad as it may sound—just what you will find when you visit the villages and hamlets. With your Indian background you should know what I mean."

I said indeed I did know and that cooking and garbage smells were the least of my concerns.

Later in the morning, with the last of the first group of outpatients attended to, I went through the ward with Eleanora.

The first patient we came to was an old man. Both his eyes were covered by bandages and he lay, unmoving, as if life were slowly ebbing from him. Eleanora assured me, however, that he was recuperating very well.

"Dr. Dick did an entropion on him last week—the old gentleman is coming along just fine." Eleanora said.

An entropion, I knew, is a condition in which the outer edge of the eyelid turns inward, causing the lashes to rub on the surface of the eye itself. It is quite often caused by trachoma, which leaves scar tissue on the underside of the eyelid. An operation to release it is frequently necessary. This condition is common in many parts of Asia and Africa. Dr. Dick had by now become a skilled eye surgeon and had done many entropions at the Chan-Y-Vien.

The rest of the patients seemed to be quite comfortable. They were chatting with their personal attendants in that quiet singsong Vietnamese which sounded so musical compared to the harsh tones of English. And while Eleanora gave instructions to Mimmie, I filled my ears and eyes.

Eleanora beckoned for me to follow her and then we both went into the clinic.

Until noon I sat beside the interviewing desk and watched and listened while the sick and injured passed before us. As

long as I've been exposed to people in need of medical care
—and that's been since my early childhood—I've never been
able to overcome the sadness I feel each time I see someone
whose health has been seriously damaged. How often I've
envied those nurses and doctors who, with remarkable self-
control, are able to treat illness without becoming emotionally involved with the patient. How much easier it must be
for them. There have been too many troubled nights when
the apparition of a man in pain, or a woman wracked with
fear, or a child confused and alienated by disease thrust
itself into my dreams.

The Chan-Y-Vien patients came into the reception room
one by one, meek, expectant, some in pain, some merely
uncomfortable, all troubled by things of the body their
minds couldn't understand. Among them were the young
woman and infant I had seen the day before waiting to be
examined during the afternoon clinic. When she had seen
them yesterday, Eleanora, with a practiced eye, had observed, "It's the mother, not the baby, who's sick. The baby
was suckling when we came in, and sick babies usually
refuse to nurse." She was right. The woman was complaining
of a cough and, because she suspected tuberculosis, Eleanora
wanted a sputum test to confirm the diagnosis.

Experience had also taught her to take advantage of the
presence of an infant. This one had probably never been
seen by a trained medical worker. But since it was then
growing late, she asked the mother to return for morning
clinic. Then we could examine the infant as well as take the
mother to the Institute Pasteur in town, in whose labora-
tories the sputum test could be performed.

Now she told Mimmie to instruct the mother to remove
the baby's cap. She said it was probably hiding a scabrous
scalp and, sure enough, the little one's head was encrusted

with sores, some of them bleeding. Under Eleanora's direction, Mimmie told the mother she would be given a salve which would heal the scabs, provided the cap was permanently discarded.

"This cap business," Eleanora explained, "is the result of an ancient taboo. You'll often find children absolutely naked but with their heads covered like this. And time and time again you'll find the same kind of scalp condition underneath.

"Unfortunately, as soon as she gets home, the mother will probably put the cap back on, without washing it, and the ointment will be of no use."

But her actions gave cause for a more optimistic prognosis than her words did. She placed a clean diaper over the child's head as a replacement for the cap and had Mimmie gently tell the mother to wash the diaper daily. Then she asked her to wait for us, as we would be going into Nhatrang and could drive her there.

We continued examining the clinic patients. Those with serious conditions would remain to see the doctor. Most were treated and sent home. It was a morning I will always remember, the first of hundreds that would provide a parade of poverty and near-futility.

They would come with cramps of the stomach, with ulcerous sores on every part of the body, with tropical fevers, with eye trouble, ear trouble, tooth trouble. Some had deep wounds that refused to heal, others would bleed from some unknown cause. I saw severe malnutrition, cases of worms and rickets, mastoids, strep throats, and, all too often, symptoms of tuberculosis. Lack of sanitation and improper nutrition were reflected in almost every case. And bodies weakened by conditions that had existed for centuries were often too fragile to combat the simplest infections.

During clinic hours I had a chance to observe Mimmie, who was remarkably efficient and considerate. When the noon break came, I took her aside. Would she, I asked, consider taking me on as a student in Vietnamese? I was determined to learn the language as quickly as possible. Not being able to communicate directly with the patients was a handicap I had to overcome.

Mimmie was delighted. "Of course. Every morning we can speak and learn. My father, Pastor Tin, has printed a small conversation book. We can start with that."

We agreed to get together for my first lesson at six-thirty the next morning. When I protested that it might be too early for her, she insisted that it was not.

"No, no. If you wish to study, I am very happy to help. Any time."

And that was the start of a wonderful friendship. I had liked her instantly and now, I was pleased to discover, she had the same reaction to me.

After lunch Eleanora had hospital business to transact on Doc Loc, Nhatrang's main shopping street. So we drove off with Mimmie and the mother and child just before two o'clock. At this hour—the equivalent of the Latin siesta—the city's streets were practically deserted. White canvas awnings hung down over many of the open-front shops and stalls to shield them from the glare of the sun. But the shops were still open for business.

We parked the Land-Rover and directed the woman to the Institute Pasteur, telling her to meet us near the car when she was finished. Then we started walking, the only people in evidence on Doc Loc—except for the Vietnamese, Chinese, and Indian shopkeepers in the shadowy darkness of their stalls.

Our first stop, because of my curiosity, was at a Chinese

medicine shop. Peering into the gloom of the interior, I noticed the balding Chinese proprietor serving two elderly customers at a wooden counter. He poured amber-colored liquid into thimble-sized cups. The customers downed it instantly, put money on the counter, and slipped out of the shadows into the sunshine.

Eleanora told me that every time she came by this store she happened to see a similar transaction. She said she thought the customers were imbibing medicine for "weakness" and suspected that they derived instant therapeutic benefit because of the draft's high alcoholic content.

We walked in to look around. The proprietor took no notice of us. Behind the counter was a motley collection of jars and bottles, all clouded by age, sweaty hands, and dust blown in from the street. These containers held what appeared to be dried fish, bits of bone, shriveled flower pods and beans, various colored powders, and liquids of many colors. There was a strong smell of peppermint which, Eleanora explained, came from small vials of oil of wintergreen. This was much prized by the Vietnamese, who resorted to it as a cureall for every possible external ailment. After it in popularity came a mahogany-colored grease which, Eleanora said, stuck to the skin like glue.

"You'll find most patients reek of peppermint and many are slathered with that brown grease. Scrub as you will, you can't remove either the smell or the goo."

As we continued down the street, Eleanora remarked that most native medicines were of ancient origin and that many fetched fantastic prices, particularly ground tiger whiskers, toenails and teeth. Tiger remedies were regarded as cures for impotence and infertility and were also used as aphrodisiacs.

We came to a Western-style drugstore. The owner, Mr.

Doi, welcomed us. A man more than twice my age, he was a little more than half my size. Eleanora and Mimmie introduced me, and he said it was a pleasure to meet the new nurse and he hoped I would favor him with trade.

Then Eleanora ordered rubbing alcohol, cans of powered boric acid, and epsom salts. Mr. Doi hastened to wrap the articles. While we waited, I asked Mimmie to tell me how to say goodbye to him.

"You say *chào*," she instructed, " which means hello, goodbye, and many other things. It is a basic word in our language and a good one to learn first." She pronounced it like the Italian *ciao*. Then she continued. "The proper way to say goodbye to a man is *chao ong*." She spelled it for me, explaining that an "n" followed by a "g" at the end of a word is pronounced "m."

As we parted, I ventured to say "*Chao ong*," and Mr. Doi beamed. He asked me to come often and promised to teach me the names of drugs in Vietnamese.

Our next stop was a shop on the other side of the city square, where Eleanora had to call for an altered dress. I waited outside with Mimmie. The dressmaker's establishment was next to an imposing building that displayed a large picture of Premier Ngo Dinh Diem. Mimmie explained that this was the government's information office. She said people, mostly from Saigon, distributed propaganda literature that told about the Premier's effort to win the war and what citizens could do to help.

A metal frame in front of the building held a movie screen for nighttime showings of films. Mimmie said men and women, when out for an evening stroll, would pause and watch the motion pictures, and the propaganda films attracted huge crowds as everyone loves a movie no matter what the subject.

33

"There is already too much war and too much politics," she said.

She had never known a time without war, nor a time when her country was without foreign soldiers. First there were the Japanese; Mimmie had been born during the Second World War. Then the French returned, a colonial power trying to regain control. Now the Americans had come to help in the defense against invaders from the north. And through it all, Vietnamese had fought other Vietnamese.

I told Mimmie that I felt deep sympathy for the Vietnamese caught in this struggle, that I had come solely for the purpose of helping heal the sick and saving lives. She said she knew this and thanked me.

Just then Eleanora came out of the dressmaker's and we walked back to the Land-Rover.

The woman was waiting for us. We drove her back to the road that led to her home, and Eleanora had Mimmie tell her to come to clinic in a week to find out the results which the Institute Pasteur would send us. At that time we could begin treatment if necessary.

Then we hastened back to the Chan-Y-Vien. The afternoon was to be a busy one. A doctor from the dispensary at the nearby U.S. Army base was scheduled to do a special procedure on a patient in our ward, when the afternoon clinic was over.

The patient was a Vietnamese boy whose uncle was a shopkeeper in town. About two weeks before, when the doctor was running some errands, the uncle had told him about his nephew. He had examined the boy briefly in the shop, decided he needed medical care and, putting the boy in his jeep, had brought him to the Chan-Y-Vien.

But neither he nor Dr. Dick was able to make a definite diagnosis. They suspected that a previous bout with beri-

34

beri, combined with generalized poor nutrition, was a factor. But it seemed that there was an accumulation of fluid in the pericardium—the sac or membrane that surrounds the heart. It was exerting pressure on the heart, preventing it from functioning normally. This condition is known as cardiac tamponade.

Immediately after the clinic we went into the operating room. The army doctor, a rangy young major in fatigues, was already bending over the Vietnamese boy.

He looked up just long enough to see who we were and then began instructing us. He explained that he was going to aspirate the pericardial sac with a suction syringe to draw off whatever fluid—it might be pus, blood, or water—had built up in it. He gave Eleanora some orders and then went to speak to the boy's uncle. Through the door I could hear his sympathetic and patient words, translated by Mimmie.

I took the boy's pulse and felt only an uneven and very faint throbbing. There was probably only a slender chance that this thin critically ill youngster would survive.

Dr. Dick joined us and the major returned. Now the operation would start. Eleanora was setting out the necessary equipment, giving me a chance to become familiar with my surroundings. I looked around, trying to absorb everything in a minute, so I could make myself useful if necessary.

The white tile walls and floors were immaculate. The same powerful overhead light that could be found in thousands of operating rooms back home was suspended over the operating table. An air conditioner set into one of the walls made the room pleasantly cool. But the white metal operating table was at least fifty years old. And the sterilizer was a pressure cooker, kept in the clinic and used for all of the Chan-Y-Vien's instruments. The equipment, including instruments, was minimal by comparison with that of Columbia Presbyterian. But the clean, cool room was to become for me a pleasantly antiseptic sanctuary, the only place in the hospital where I could pursue my duties away from the gaze of curious onlookers.

While the doctors scrubbed at the sink in the adjoining scrub room I shook powder into their rubber surgical gloves. I held the gloves up while they worked their fingers into them.

Quickly but deftly the Army surgeon explored the external region of the patient's heart by tapping his chest. Then, spreading an area of skin taut, he held his other hand out for the hypodermic syringe. Slowly and carefully he inserted the needle through the skin and then deeper, aspirating every few millimeters to see if the fluid in the sac had been reached.

For a mere fraction of a second a flush of color came to the boy's face. Then, suddenly, the frail body shuddered and became still. Instantly the major withdrew the needle. The boy's heart had stopped beating. There was no pulse, no murmur of a heartbeat, no life. Immediately he began to massage the child's chest with his strong hands. Oblivious to what surrounded him, he worked as if his own life depended on the outcome.

Time seemed to have become suspended. Except for the air conditioner, the only sound in the room was the heavy breathing of the Army doctor. Beads of perspiration formed on his forehead and neck as he rubbed firmly on the inert little chest. Finally, after ten minutes of silent battle with death, he sadly gave up.

The doctor made a final examination of the boy. He slowly removed his gloves. Eleanora laid a sheet over the wasted body. I felt quite numb. Even though I knew there had been little hope for the boy, the suddenness of his death left me in shock.

Eleanora came over and put her hand on my arm. "I know this has upset you," she said kindly. "I think we all feel the same way. I'm sure you know that no doctor or nurse ever takes the death of a patient easily." I did know that. But her words made me feel somewhat better.

She suggested that it might be best if I returned to the house. She told me she would clean up and arrange for the transfer of the boy's body to the car. Then she would take the uncle home.

I was about to leave the hospital when I heard the Army doctor speaking to the uncle.

"Are you certain this gentleman understands that we did everything possible to save the boy?" the doctor asked Mimmie.

"He understands. He says to thank you very much for all your effort. Mr. Ky knew from talking to you before that the chance was small."

I stared at the man. He looked as though he were carved of wax. In time I would get used to this typical expression of stoicism when confronted with inevitable misfortune. But this was my first exposure to the Vietnamese reaction to death, and I ached with sympathy for the man and his family.

In order to have something to do, to take my mind off what I had just seen, I went into the ward. Patients were talking and their family attendants were moving about. Mimmie followed me quickly and explained that the ward had learned of the boy's death. She told me that if he had died in the ward, those patients whose beds were near his would have moved to other beds, to avoid the spirit that would wander until he was buried. I asked what would happen if we needed those beds, or the boy's for that matter, and she explained that the taboo only affected those who had known the boy. New patients coming in next day would not be bothered by his spirit.

Eleanora came in then. Dr. Dick had decided to take the truck bearing the body into town himself.

As we left the ward, we heard the engine of the Land-Rover starting up. The patients and their attendants scurried to the windows, and my last view of the ward that evening was of a dozen faces peering out, with more curiosity than sympathy, as the truck left to carry the dead boy home. And somehow, although I was still shaken, I felt a little more prepared for what lay before me.

4

THREE WEEKS HAD gone by when Dr. Hasselblad, my father, arrived in Nhatrang. As president of the American Leprosy Missions he was on an inspection visit to Asian leprosariums. I had known, before I left home, that Dad's visit to Vietnam would follow closely on the heels of my own arrival. Yet it seemed that I had hardly settled in, had hardly even had a chance to think of home, when we were reunited.

It was good to see Dad, even better than I had imagined it would be. I had become so involved in the Chan-Y-Vien, in my lessons in Vietnamese, and adjusting to the routine of the hospital that I had little time to relax and think about anything other than day-to-day problems.

The morning Dad arrived in Nhatrang he, Dr. Dick and I set off in the Land-Rover for the Banmethuot leprosarium, 180 miles from Nhatrang. I had looked forward to this trip as a pleasant change of pace for me, a relaxed outing into the countryside. But it was not exactly that.

Tailgating the Land-Rover from the time we left Nhatrang was a large flatbed truck filled with Vietnamese soldiers. Government officials in Saigon had urged my father to accept an armed escort.

They explained that there had been numerous Vietcong raids on hamlets near Banmethuot; houses had been burned, crops destroyed, and village officials kidnapped.

The uneasiness I felt at being followed by a virtual arsenal of weapons was only slightly eased by Dr. Dick's conviction that the rifles weren't loaded. He had noted that none of the soldiers wore cartridge belts and assumed that headquarters had probably forgotten to issue ammunition. But from their appearance of extreme youth and their general air of uneasiness, I judged the soldiers to be new recruits, which meant that in case of trouble their presence might prove more dangerous to us than their absence. I was therefore relieved when we finally arrived at the town of Banmethuot with about five miles to go to the leprosarium and our escort left us. Their orders, apparently, were to go no further.

The last leg of the trip was unbelievable. We could have walked faster than we drove and been considerably safer. The trail—for this was what the road narrowed to—was incredibly bad, filled with ruts and potholes. Almost as soon as we left the town we were in a jungly rain forest dense with tropical growth. The wooden bridges which spanned the streams creaked and sagged under the weight of the Land-Rover.

We inched the car along for what seemed like hours. The vegetation had been burned on both sides of the road so no sniper could hide there. I thought that, if we had so much difficulty getting just one vehicle through, it would surely be impossible to move a large motorized military unit and its equipment over such a road. And I wondered if Vietcong guerrillas lay hidden in the underbrush, watching us go by. It seemed ironic that we had lost our escort just before coming to what could have been the most dangerous part of the journey.

Finally we came to the leprosarium, set in a clearing cut out of the lush growth. Since it served members of the Rhadde tribe primarily—which lived in the Banmethuot area and for some reason has a high incidence of leprosy— most of its houses were of the usual tribal construction. They were made of bamboo and raised above the ground on wooden stilts, a style of building that obviously served to keep them high and dry above the kind of jungle tangle we had just driven through. These were the patients' cottages. The administration and hospital buildings were of more usual and permanent construction.

We were greeted by Dr. Ardel Vietti, the woman who operated the hospital. My father told her of our armed escort to the town of Banmethuot. But Dr. Vietti told us that our lone arrival was a blessing in disguise, since the presence of armed men at the leprosarium might stir the Vietcong to retaliate. "The road in here has a thousand eyes," she said. "We know that Vietcong lookouts report back on every move we make. We have no idea why we should be under surveillance, but we make a special point of never violating our peaceful purpose in this area. The arrival of one man with a rifle, let alone a truckload of soldiers, could have resulted in a raid. At the very least they would have placed mines along the only road leading in here."

Dr. Vietti also said that the heavy truck and its load might have weighed too much for any one of the bridges. If a bridge had collapsed, the leprosarium would have been isolated for some time, until the slow-moving Vietnamese government got around to fixing it.

Dr. Vietti was an energetic and dedicated woman, and her kindness impressed me immediately. I had observed leprosy in India—both its medical and social aspects. But this visit reaffirmed after many years the tragedy that is it's victim's lot.

Man has always feared that which he could not understand and leprosy, throughout recorded history, has been one of the most deeply feared of human diseases. Although there are probably more than fifteen million people throughout the world, including the United States, afflicted with this superstition-shrouded disabling disease, only a small percentage receive any kind of treatment. Leprosy today can be treated, and in most cases arrested, but so far there has been little success in treating the society which regards the leprosy patient as an object of dread, an unclean being cursed by his God.

As I visited the wards and houses where the patients lived, it was not so much their physical disabilities that disturbed me as it was their emotional withdrawal, their fear of causing revulsion.

Since I spoke so few Vietnamese words at that time, and was in complete ignorance of the Rhadde language, I was silent during the first part of my visit. But I soon became aware that my muteness was being misconstrued. The patients would turn away from us, afraid for their scars and mutilations to be seen. I would not have had these people think that I was too horrified to speak so, with my very limited Vietnamese vocabulary, I stopped to chat with some of them.

The change in attitude was immediate. Faces that had been hidden now looked up with interest, indicating a welcome. Rejected by their own people, they appreciated the small gesture of friendship I was able to make.

Medical treatment and nursing care were available to them but it would take much more than drugs and surgery to give them even the slightest sense of normal life. The stigma that centuries of superstition attached to their illness had driven all hope from them. Because nothing could erase the horror with which their countrymen viewed them, they would continue to be relegated to isolation villages deep in the jungle.

I realized that it would take a great deal of strength to nurse in a leprosarium. I had thought that I could handle or cope with any kind of illness. But what I saw that day so filled me with despair that I doubted that I could ever return.

Later, over dinner, I spoke with the hospital staff. The five nurses, like the doctor in charge, were deeply committed to working with leprosy. They seemed intelligent, sensitive, and apparently indefatigable in their efforts to rehabilitate their patients. The young American man who handled all the maintenance chores at the leprosarium was a paxman. Paxmen are conscientious objectors of draft age who, because of religious scruples, refuse to serve in the military. The American government permits them to enlist with the Mennonite Central Committee to work in voluntary service for the time they would otherwise serve in the armed forces. They can be found serving all over the world in all kinds of situations and institutions.

Soon the night noises of the jungle signaled that the day was over. It had been a long, intense one for me. For the others, it had been just one more round in their persistent battle.

Next morning after breakfast we left the leprosarium and

headed back through the jungle. The going was no easier than it had been the day before. By late afternoon I was again at the airport with my father. Although we had spent much time together, we hadn't really had a chance to be alone to talk. He studied me carefully now as we sat over coffee in the airport café. I knew he was making mental notes of what to tell the family about me. The creases along his forehead indicated concern.

Finally he spoke, part father, part physician. "Marva, you look tired. You've lost weight and underneath that beautiful tan you look wan and drawn. Is there anything bothering you—the people you're working with, the climate, the load of work on your shoulders?"

I quickly reassured him that everything was wonderful and that I was overjoyed with my job. But I don't think he believed me. The truth was that I didn't quite believe it myself.

My father warned me about overworking once the patient load increased. He was absolutely certain that it would grow since he believed that it was just a question of time before the local Vietnamese would accept and trust what we were doing. I was still not quite sure. But his loving confidence in me buoyed me that afternoon. As he boarded the plane I felt a renewed vigor.

Soon afterward Eleanora Weaver left the Chan-Y-Vien to return to the States, the end of her term of service. Now I was on my own. Much as I was anxious to handle everything by myself, I regretted that I could no longer rely on her three years of experience in South Vietnam.

My first test came almost immediately. While we were at dinner there was a rap at the door. Linh, one of our young patients, stood outside gesturing frantically.

Linh was scheduled for corrective eye surgery next day

and was supposed to be resting in the ward. Only an emergency would cause her to disregard the doctor's orders.

In pantomime, because she spoke no English, she indicated a swollen abdomen, moved as if in pain and then pointed to the hospital. What she was very clearly conveying to us was that a pregnant woman, probably in labor, had come to the hospital.

We found the young woman waiting for us in the reception room, rocking back and forth on her heels, rubbing her large abdomen. It was obvious that she was in great pain but she never once cried out or indicated her discomfort by any of the traditional labor contortions common among Western women.

Throughout the time I was in Vietnam, I rarely saw hysteria in a woman in labor. Those who came to the hospital to deliver their babies usually came at the very end of their labor and generally arrived alone. Although they were built small, they always seemed in full control of their labor. I noticed many of the women using breathing techniques similar to what is being taught to American women in natural childbirth classes.

Dr. Dick helped the young mother—she appeared to be in her late teens—into the operating room and then I prepared her for an examination. The doctor told me the baby would be breech and that he might need high forceps for the delivery. But since the woman was still in early labor it would probably be some time before the infant would be born.

Mimmie came in then, alerted by Linh that we might need her. She learned from the patient that three previous children had died at birth and that this delivery would be premature, since she was only in the seventh month of pregnancy.

I looked at the delicate young thing and wondered at her

stoicism in the face of such a history. I thought it was quite unlikely that I, or any American woman I knew, could remain silent and completely self-contained when faced with such an ordeal.

Although I wanted to linger by her side, there were more important things to be done. In the first place, I had to figure out a way to sterilize the forceps the doctor had ordered. Our pressure cooker-sterilizer was too small to hold them. It finally occurred to me to use one of the hospital's metal washdrums. I routed out the night watchman and between us we filled the large drum and set it over an open fire behind the hospital.

It took the better part of an hour to bring the water to a boil but finally it was done and the sterile forceps were brought to the operating room. During this time I must have been in and out of the operating room over a dozen times, offering my assistance, trying to keep track of a multitude of things at once.

After a while it became clear that it would be several hours before the woman would be ready to deliver. Dr. Dick and I decided to take turns sleeping and so he set up a cot in the room we used as a laboratory while I remained in the delivery room.

For half the night I stood beside the operating table supporting the young mother, making her as comfortable as possible, since stabbing back pains prevented her from lying flat. By an effective but simple sign language she and I communicated throughout the long wait. In this way I learned of her anxiety about returning home without a child to present to her husband. Although he hadn't come along with her to the hospital—Vietnamese men, according to an ancient taboo, must never be in the proximity of birth—he was worried about her and very anxious to have a son.

As the hours stretched into morning, we changed positions several times. For a while she squatted on a pad I had placed on the floor while I sat facing her, my legs crossed under me. It occurred to me that we would have presented a strange spectacle in a Western hospital.

Finally, at three A.M., an examination showed that the woman was almost fully dilated and would deliver soon. Dr. Dick came in.

Agonizing minutes later, a tiny boy was born, followed immediately by another infant, a twin to the first.

As I handled these fragile babies I realized that they would probably not live out the hour. They were simply too small, too weak to face life outside their mother's womb. After the doctor finished with the mother he came to look at the infants. But I could see little hope on his face. Soon, first the older, then the younger, died as they lay side by side in the bamboo baby basket.

I thought of the hospital facilities that were commonplace at home but completely unavailable here. If we only had incubators and the other equipment necessary for premature birth, they might have had some chance. But with only the simplest and most basic equipment on hand, it was impossible to save lives such as these.

The young woman knew without being told that she was still childless and an expression of utter weariness and defeat crossed her face. I carried her into the darkened ward and placed her in a bed apart from the others. As I was leaving her she groped for my arm.

I returned to the operating room, grateful for the hard physical work that had to be done. First I wrapped the small, still bodies in cloth and placed them in the basket. Their father would come next morning to take them to the home they never knew. Then, because only a woman could,

47

or would, perform these tasks, I cleaned up the room, scrubbed the floor, and washed out the sheets, with Mimmie's help.

The dawn had already come up when I returned to the silent bungalow. It had been a long night and I was both emotionally and physically exhausted. As I crawled into bed the haunted eyes of the disappointed woman were before me. But I fell asleep instantly.

An hour later my alarm clock wakened me. It was almost the clinic hour and I couldn't afford the luxury of sleeping until noon. But, strangely, that short sleep had fully refreshed me and, except for the rings under my eyes, I felt no different from any other morning.

That afternoon Linh underwent the second operation on her malformed eyelid, with Dr. Dick and the Army doctor performing the delicate surgery.

Although I had known Linh only a short time and we were not yet able to speak together in Vietnamese, we had developed a remarkable rapport. I knew that for the past two years following the infection of her eyelid she had avoided having surgery and instead chose to bear her discomfort in silence. When Dr. Dick came to the Chan-Y-Vien he tried without success to win her permission for corrective surgery. Finally, when failing vision almost forced her to give up her work as a seamstress she consented.

The Army major who performed the operation was a fine surgeon and I particularly looked forward to watching him. Unlike the ordeal of the previous night, this was a quick, efficient and stimulating experience. And Linh went through it beautifully.

Afterward, the job of returning the operating room to order again fell on my shoulders. The Army major was appalled that I should be responsible for such work.

I explained to him that, if I didn't do it, it simply wouldn't get done since the men avoided the operating room because it was also the scene of childbirth. When he suggested that I find a female to do the job, I wondered why that hadn't occurred to me before. Although eventually I would get a woman to do the bulk of this work, there would still be many times when the chief nurse would double as scrubwoman.

Now the doctor insisted that I leave the work for the time being and take a much needed airing. For the first time in many weeks I felt free and female for a few hours. He waited while I put on a fresh summer dress and fixed my hair. I felt fine as I anticipated my first evening out. It was just the tonic I needed.

We dined on lobster, toured a local fishing village, bargained unsuccessfully for a boat for him, and we talked and laughed, forgetting for a time the grimmer realities of our lives.

5

"IT'S TIME WE looked into the situation of the tribespeople at Phuoc Luong," Rudi Lichti announced. He had just come from Saigon for a meeting with the hospital's board of directors and also to look into the necessity of sending relief supplies of food to the tribal villages.

There were twelve hundred tribesmen living about sixteen miles away, in the valley beyond Nhatrang. But not many of them had come to the Chan-Y-Vien for care. Mr. Lichti felt that we should inspect the conditions at their crowded village. Much to my delight he asked me to join him for this trip.

And so, once again, I was in the Land-Rover heading into the countryside. As he drove, Mr. Lichti gave some background on what I would find. The area we were going into was a resettlement village in the lowlands designated by the

South Vietnamese government for the mountain people who had taken refuge from the Vietcong.

He said I would find them very different from the Vietnamese I had already encountered. They have different racial characteristics. Their skin is darker and they are bigger boned. They are also more primitive. But they are a friendly, happy, and hardworking people.

The circumstances which had brought these tribes to Phuoc Luong were being repeated throughout South Vietnam. Their villages, scattered over the hillsides, were self-sufficient units, and therefore they had had very little contact with the lowland people. When the Vietcong came into their area their entire tribal way of life was upset. The Vietcong had asked for their allegiance, to be proved by the regular provision of food and fighting men. But these tribesmen had refused to cooperate, wanting nothing to do with the outsiders and unwilling to alter their lives for a cause they neither understood nor cared about.

In retaliation the Vietcong started a series of raids on the tribal villages, burning homes and crops and kidnapping young men and elders. Finally, with their means of sustenance destroyed and their social units disrupted, the tribal people were forced to leave their homeland.

The people now at Phuoc Luong had walked more than two hundred miles through hazardous mountain trails. Most of them, like refugees everywhere, had taken only what they could carry; for the women this meant their young children and the clothes they wore on their backs. And there were those who had to be left behind—too sick, weak, or old to undertake the long trip.

When they arrived in Phuoc Luong they had no shelter and no food. The South Vietnam government allocated land and some food supplies to these displaced people, but the supplies were insufficient and the land was so poor that no South Vietnamese could have lived on it. For these refugees, however, it was home. They planted their fields and waited for their first harvest.

At the time of our visit they were still waiting for that first harvest, after eight months and their third planting. The first crop had died because of the poor land, and the Vietcong had reappeared and destroyed the second crop. Rudi Lichti had been sending bulgur wheat, enough for four days out of every seven. To buy food for the other three days, the people cut and sold wood to the surrounding Vietnamese villages.

As we drove into the village the signs of poverty and deprivation were everywhere. There were no streets, just hard-packed dirt paths which turned into a sea of mud when it rained. The houses were primitive, providing totally inadequate protection against sun, wind and rain. The young children were naked except for some ornaments, and too many had the spindly bowed legs and distended abdomens characteristic of severe malnutrition. And even the few animals I saw in the area looked as if they hadn't been fed in months.

Yet the reception we received did not make me think of a hungry, desperate people. The men met us with wide grins and clustered around the jeep to greet us. The women, after they had hurried indoors to cover their bare breasts, were as cordial to us as their menfolk.

For a moment I thought I was back in India. The scraggly animals, the elaborate jewelry and long, wraparound skirts of the women, the coloring and facial structure of the children, the open, wood-fed hearths over which they cooked—these all reminded me of the villages I had known.

But there were some very significant differences. For one thing, there were four rather crude Protestant churches and one Catholic church. I was told that 85 per cent were Christians and that their religion, an odd combination of Western and native beliefs, played an important role in their lives.

The village had been constructed as a fortress—and a rather ingenious and effective one at that. Since there was just a handful of firearms among the entire community they had devised other deterrents to attack. Surrounding the entire village were two high fences constructed of sharply pointed poles placed side by side. Between was a dirt embankment planted with a sharp bamboo spikes. Alongside each house was an underground shelter to be used by the women and children in the event of an attack. I later learned that the relocation villages throughout South Vietnam were similarly protected.

I marvelled at the persistence of these people in keeping out the Vietcong. It was only later, when I got to know them better, that I understood that any effort from almost any group to disrupt their centuries-old way of life would have met with the same stalwart resistance.

The Vietnamese pastor who was our guide and translator pointed out the enormous piles of rocks inside the bamboo fence. When the Vietcong had first attempted to raid the village five months before, they had been turned away by villagers hurling these rocks at them. Between the rocks and the spikes the raiders were never able to get close enough to the fence to break through.

As we walked through the village the pastor spoke of his particular concern about the lack of medical care. Rudi told him that we hoped we would be able to come again with complete medical facilities now that the Vietcong raids had tapered off. I hoped also that we would be able to get some of these people, who so obviously needed our services, to come to the Chan-Y-Vien.

The pastor smiled his gratitude and then turned to the large group of people who had been following us throughout our walk. When he held up his hand the group instantly became silent, all eyes turning to him and us.

Then he translated our promise into the various tribal languages of the resettlement village. Although the tribes people are not usually demonstrative, his words brought an instant response of gratitude directed at Mr. Lichti and myself.

After a hurried conference in a group gathered near us, one young man stepped forward. He wore tattered shorts and rubber sandals wrought out of a discarded tire, and he had the drawn look of someone who has eaten very little over a long time. But in his hands he held a cluster of bananas, which he extended to us as a gift.

Although he knew that the donors could make much better use of this present than we could, Mr. Lichti accepted it with the graciousness with which it was given. After our visit was over we talked about the supplies we would need to fill the Land-Rover for its day's work as a mobile medical unit at Phuoc Luong. Rudi planned to have Dr. Dick return to Saigon with him for the necessary supplies.

One morning about a month later Dr. Dick, Pastor Pham Xuam Tin, two of the male hospital staff, and I were in the Land-Rover heading to Phuoc Luong. Pastor Tin, a member of the Protestant Church Council, was president of the Chan-Y-Vien's board of directors and, on this trip, interpreter.

With this visit we all hoped to lay the foundation for a long and effective relationship between the tribespeople and the hospital. We had learned that one of the International Voluntary Service workers had provided a fund to cover the travel expenses of those who needed care and would come by Lambretta to the hospital. To cover the expenses for their return transportation and also to provide food for them while they were there, Dr. and Mrs. Dick provided a similar fund at the hospital boosted by special contributions from friends at home.

When we arrived at Phuoc Luong a crowd of more than five hundred people came out to greet us. Pastor Tin conducted a short service and then informed the crowd why we were there.

Dr. Dick set up our makeshift clinic in the village school house. I had brought along a folding table and the villagers supplied benches for each of us and our interpreters.

And then we began. In three hours we saw and treated 220 patients, working with lightening speed. We dressed uncounted numbers of severe tropical ulcers. We gave dozens of penicillin injections. We distributed thousands and thousands of pills, most of the multivitamins. Our interpreters explained their use over and over and over. Dr. Dick pulled at least a dozen infected teeth. I listened to several dozen fetal heart beats. And we knew that a few months of eating nourishing and plentiful food would all but eliminate ninety per cent of the ailments we encountered.

The next time Rudolph Lichti came to the Chan-Y-Vien, his wife Elda and their teen-aged son Martin were with him. The Dicks were away for a few days and the Lichtis stayed with me in the bungalow. Rudi had more relief supplies for the Phuoc Luong villagers.

On this second trip I personally saw 210 people. Fortunately, most of the cases were minor and I was able to handle them without a physician's assistance. The number of cases of diarrhea had risen alarmingly; but there were no real crises. Unfortunately I wasn't yet able to handle dental problems. Before long I would find an Army dentist to teach me how to extract badly decayed teeth, a skill that would be as much a boon to my work at the hospital as in the field.

On our way home we decided to stop and examine an old deserted French fort. But when we arrived we discovered that the dilapidated structure had been appropriated by a refugee mountain tribe and that most of those in this group were ill.

The situation at this fort was much more desperate than at the resettlement village. The tribe of about 65 people was completely destitute. They had arrived just the week before and so far had had to fend for themselves. Mr. Lichti made an inventory of what was needed, so he could deliver supplies within the week. I took note of the obvious medical needs of these people. When we left, the image of them standing around to see us off was so moving that I found I couldn't look back. It was good to return home that day.

I had looked forward to Easter as sort of the first milestone during my tour of duty. On the morning of Easter Sunday we all attended a sunrise service on the beach. It was conducted by the chaplain from the U.S. Army base that had been set up in Nhatrang not far from the 8th Field Hospital. As the dawn came up over our small congregation and the sky filled with a wide array of glorious colors, I joined in prayer and song with a lightheartedness I had felt too infrequently in the past months. It was comforting to observe this day in much the same way I had observed it since I was a child. But it saddened me somewhat to see that our congregation was entirely made up of Americans, most of them soldiers.

Later that morning I attended a devotional service at a Vietnamese Christian chapel. On this occasion I was one of only a few Caucasians. But I was welcomed as warmly as if I were one of their own people. What I found particularly interesting was that the service completely bypassed the fact that this was Easter. I had noted the same thing the previous Sunday, which was Palm Sunday. Even though Christianity was a significant bond between many of the Vietnamese people and those here from the West, centuries of history and traditions had had their effect on its practice.

I regarded that Easter Sunday as the end of my novitiate.

6

My PROGRESS WITH the Vietnamese language was proceeding well. In the early morning Mimmie and I would go into the quiet, deserted doctor's office of the hospital and work from the book written by her father. During the day, beginning in clinic when Mimmie translated back and forth between the patients, the staff workers, and myself, I would repeat aloud what she had said. I found that the more I repeated, the more I remembered. Since everyone knew that I was trying to break the language barrier, they all made an effort to speak slowly in my presence.

Although still unable to ask patients questions, I could understand a good part of their conversation. Because speaking the language involves the use of a complicated singsong technique, with different intonations for the same word indicating different meanings, I would often use the right word but impart to it the wrong meaning as a result of articulating it at the wrong tone level.

Linh, the young girl who had undergone eye surgery, and I were now good friends. Since she shared my delight in the beauty of the beach down at the cove, she often joined me late in the day when I had a free hour. Speaking slowly she would tell me the names of things we would pass—flowers, trees, birds, sea objects. Often she brought fruit along for us to share as we climbed over rocks and walked along the sand. A favorite of hers, which in time I came to enjoy, was green guavas flavored with a mixture of chopped chili peppers and salt.

I now also had a bicycle, which gave me just a little bit of extra freedom in my hours off. At the time I was planning to buy it, I knew a sharp bargainer would be needed, and so I enlisted the services of Anh Ba, the hospital laundryman. One afternoon he came to me and announced that he had finally found the right bicycle, at the right price, and asked me to come with him to examine it. I went, I looked, and I bought a beautiful white bicycle in exactly the condition Anh Ba had described. The problem then arose as to what I should wear while riding it. Mimmie and Linh were concerned that I be properly dressed, which meant protecting my legs against exposure above the knees. Finally they suggested that Linh make me a pair of knee-length knickers to be worn under my full skirts. "If a fast wind comes and blows the skirt, you'll be decent," they concurred.

To find just the right fabric we all made an expedition to the open markets in Nhatrang. This was my first visit to the market area and I found it quite hot, the smell from the food area almost overpowering, but fascinating nevertheless. Laid out like most Asian bazaars, each stall just a few feet long and deep, it presented a wild array of colors, objects, smells and sounds.

Shopowners stood or squatted beside their wares, loudly hawking merchandise to those who passed by. While a sale was taking place the voices rose, the women invariably out-shouting the men. I had thought the Vietnamese a quiet people until now but apparently in business it was common-place to bargain loudly.

Linh drove a hard bargain with the Indian yard-goods merchant and we acquired a piece of black cloth, which would later make a pair of breeches.

When we returned to the hospital we found that two emergency cases had arrived in our absence. While Dr. Dick attended a young boy whose hand had been crushed in a sugar-cane cutter, I talked with the other patient, a pregnant woman. Questioning revealed that she was in the ninth month but had felt no fetal movement for several months. Dr. Dick concluded that her condition, which he called a missed abortion, would be likely to cause her to hemorrhage after delivery. She would need transfusions of blood plasma rich in fibrogens to stop the bleeding. This would be a major problem since neither the Chan-Y-Vien nor the Province Hospital at that time had a blood bank.

Shortly afterward her labor began. As expected, she deliv-ered a stillborn infant and then began to hemorrhage uncon-trollably. Dr. Dick, using every device at his disposal, tried vainly to halt the bleeding. Finally, in desperation, he an-nounced that we had no choice but to take her to the Prov-ince Hospital.

As we were leaving the Chan-Y-Vien, the woman lying over a thick layer of sheets and blankets on an improvised stretcher, a man emerged from the shadows. He was the husband. He had come even though it is customary for men

she had come sooner than she was expected. Later, when my Vietnamese improved, I learned that Ba'-ba's arrival had not been an accident. She had seen us drop Mimmie at her home at six in the morning and realized that there had probably been an emergency that would require her assistance.

In all the time I was to be at the Chan-Y-Vien none of my co-workers and friends was ever to prove more devoted than Ba'-ba. It was largely because she shouldered so many of the menial burdens and worked with such diligence that I could attend to so many medical chores and still maintain necessary standards of hospital cleanliness.

And so, together, we worked to wipe out the evidence of the tragedy of the past hours and to ready the Chan-Y-Vien for whatever drama the hours ahead might bring.

Later that morning, the man we had left at his wife's bedside at the Province Hospital came to tell us that in spite of the operation his wife had died. He asked for the few belongings that had been left with us. With this small bundle in hand, he would return to his family of five children and explain why their mother would not be coming home again.

7

As SPRING PROGRESSED the weather became hotter and dryer. The hills surrounding Nhatrang turned from green to brown to parched tan. The air remained still and heavy for weeks on end and the roads were covered with a deep layer of sandy dust.

Outside the Chan-Y-Vien everything seemed to slow down and become quieter. But within the hospital the pace had been increasing.

Word about the hospital and what we were doing had spread through the city and surrounding communities. The patients I had been so anxious for had finally materialized. Now attendance at morning clinics averaged 75 people, the majority of them women with children and infants. Our efforts to win the people's confidence were now paying off. It seemed that the more patients we treated, the more patients we received. Word-of-mouth advertising seemed to be responsible. Like people everywhere, the Vietnamese would shop around until they found a doctor or hospital that suited them. And one satisfied patient invariably told several others. For the first time the Chan-Y-Vien was operating at near capacity.

But with the increase in patients came problems we weren't equipped to handle. With only one physician, one nurse, and extremely limited supplies of equipment and drugs, we had to turn more and more frequently to the Army hospital. Army doctors began stopping by almost daily and were always available to us for emergency surgery. We also had to call on them increasingly for special medicines it was impossible to obtain elsewhere in Nhatrang.

To meet this new and constant demand for drugs, Dr. Dick had to make frequent trips to Saigon. This was always a frustrating affair in which he would make the rounds of Vietnamese government agencies which controlled the distribution of medicines provided by U.S. aid programs. More often than not only a fraction of his requisition was supplied. Too often the very items we needed, sent by the U.S. government or the M.C.C., would be right in Saigon, tied up in a snarl of red tape that might take weeks or even months to untangle. And we would have to resort to buying the things we needed at exorbitant prices from black marketeers who had managed to pilfer these very supplies before they reached their intended destination.

During one of Dr. Dick's trips at the end of April, I learned what was involved in running a hospital single-handed.

At the time he left there was only one serious case in the hospital. And he agreed that I could handle it with no difficulty. This was the case of the fisherman Nam, who had been operated on just two days before. Nam, supported by homemade crutches, had come to us one morning in excruciating pain. In his condition it was miraculous that he had contrived to get to the hospital with only the help of his ten-year-old son. He was unable to walk, he had a frighteningly high fever, and his pain would have immobilized almost anyone else.

But Nam had a fatalism about himself that I was often to observe among the Vietnamese. He believed he was "lucky-lucky," the literal translation of the expression which implied that it wasn't yet a man's time to succumb to death.

Dr. Dick examined the leg wound. It had been covered by a rotting bandage that was stained with seepage from a severe infection. While the doctor delicately removed the unclean dressing, which released a staggering smell of decay, Mimmie and I learned Nam's history from his son.

Three weeks before, while swimming alongside his motor-driven boat, the fisherman's ankle had been caught in the boat's propeller. There was a great deal of bleeding, and the pain was so severe that he was unable to walk. Finally, a week later he went to the Province Hospital. The ankle was dressed and he was told to return in a few days. At his second visit the doctor told him that the ankle would never heal and that it would be necessary to amputate. Nam refused to accept this verdict and left the hospital. If he lost a foot, he would not be able to swim after his nets. Now he had come to the Chan-Y-Vien in the hope that we could save his foot and thereby his livelihood.

Dr. Dick wanted the Army's orthopedic surgeon to examine the leg and two of the Army physicians came out to look at Nam. The operation performed that afternoon was a debridement—the removal of the infected tissue. It was preliminary to major surgery and took several hours but went well. It seemed likely that the foot could be saved. Nam was quite weakened by the ordeal and it would take some time for the infection to abate completely. In the meantime, while Dr. Dick would be away, he would require extensive postoperative care.

With only one patient who needed a great deal of attention I felt no uneasiness at the prospect of being left on my own for a few days. But no sooner had the doctor left than the hospital came to sudden life.

At the head of the line for morning clinic was a woman with a sick baby. A preliminary examination made me almost certain that the baby had meningitis. The Army doctors arrived that afternoon and performed a spinal tap on the infant boy, confirming my diagnosis. Then they set up the intravenous injection he required.

While they worked on the infant, an eighteen-month-old girl was brought in with massive lymphangitis—inflammation of the lymphatic vessels—which was the result of the spread of a chicken pox infection. She required large doses of penicillin, which we were able to give her.

After seeing that everything was under control the doctors left. Soon after their departure, however, the needle that had been used for the infant clotted up. It was too large for the tiny vein. I frantically tried to start the intravenous fluid running again, but that was impossible.

A note went off to the Army hospital, and again a doctor came out to help me, bringing the materials we lacked for doing a cut-down. In this procedure a piece of very thin plastic tubing is inserted into a vein, usually in the leg, and sewn in place. It is used when a traditional intravenous needle cannot be retained, and is usually necessary with children, who move about and dislodge the needle. The army doctor remained long enough to make certain that the tube was functioning and that the medication was continuing to drip properly. Then he returned to the base.

I sat by the infant's side through the long night while the

mother slept on a grass mat on the floor near the bed. But my vigil was in vain. Just before the dawn came up the child died.

There is no greater ordeal for a doctor or nurse than telling a mother her child is dead. No matter what is said, it never seems to be right. After removing the infant's body from the ward I woke the mother and led her outside. She heard me in silence, her head bowed.

I watched, sadly and helplessly, as the bereft woman gathered up her few belongings—a mat, a blanket. She wrapped the infant's body in cloth to conceal it, folding it into a bundle. Her face was set in an expression of total acceptance as she walked to the main road. She would take the body home in a *xich-lo* or Lambretta; the driver would think the package in her arms contained clothing or food. No form of public transportation would willingly carry a dead body. If an adult had died, relatives would have arranged for a coffin to be brought in, and would have bargained with the driver of a Lambretta cab or a cargo bus to transport the body. There were no funeral homes as there are in the States to take over when death comes.

After the women left I returned to the ward to clean up. The bed remained empty all that day—the other patients even avoided walking next to it for several hours. Whenever I went into the ward the empty bed reminded me of the poor dead baby and the uncomplaining grief of its mother.

And that was the way my supervision of the Chan-Y-Vien continued until Dr. Dick returned. Every day brought new crises, some small, some not so small. Every day Army doctors came by to offer and give assistance. The weekend after Dr. Dick returned, I took a short vacation, at his suggestion, and visited friends of my family in Saigon.

My next nighttime vigil was kept for an entirely different reason.

It was the night before May Day. I worked late into the evening at the hospital. And I had promised to drive a patient to her home near the city.

Mimmie tried to talk me out of going. Because of the holiday, she feared Vietcong demonstrations and felt it was unwise for anyone to be on the road. But I believed she was exaggerating the danger.

She insisted on coming along with me. She argued that I might get lost trying to find the woman's house by myself. Although I protested that it wasn't necessary I was grateful for her company.

The trip through the quiet night was completely uneventful—the streets were deserted, indicating that others were also frightened—but Mimmie remained hidden on the floor throughout the short ride. Even when I told her that no one was around, not even on a bicycle, she refused to sit up.

Although I had had no direct encounter with the Vietcong, the empty streets and Mimmie's terror suddenly made the menace seem close at hand.

The streets were still silent as we returned to the Chan-Y-Vien, and Mimmie was still afraid. I parked the Land-Rover and Mimmie went to her home, which was nearby.

The Dicks had already retired, and I went to my room. Just as I was getting ready for bed, the calm night was shattered by the sound of a violent explosion. I dashed out of my room to join Dr. and Mrs. Dick. The whole bungalow was rocking as reverberations from the explosion continued. While Mrs. Dick calmed the three children, the doctor and I speculated on the cause of the blast. The likelihood of May Day demonstrations was uppermost in our minds, but when we analyzed the direction from which the explosion seemed to have come we realized that there was another possibility.

Not too far from the Chan-Y-Vien was a Vietnamese training academy for noncommissioned officers. We had often heard the sound of tracer bullets in the evening as the soldiers practiced marksmanship. The blast seemed to come from the same direction. Friends of mine were teaching at the academy, and I was concerned for their safety. But when the sound of the explosion finally died away, and no second blast followed, we concluded that there was no real danger. Still shaken, I returned to the hospital to reassure the patients and our Vietnamese aides, who chattered agitatedly until I spoke to them. Finally I was able to get a few hours of sleep.

In the morning we learned that an accidental detonation of a quantity of TNT had produced the blast. And we discovered cracks in the walls of the bungalow, a souvenir of the night's events. But aside from the loss of sleep there were no ill effects.

Brigadier General and Mrs. Howard Eggleston, friends of my parents who had been my hosts in Saigon, came to Nhatrang for a few days to inspect the military base there. I spent some time with them, along with other Army officers, and wherever we were, whatever we were doing, inevitably the social chatter would turn to a discussion of military aspects of the war.

The number of casualties—both Vietnamese and American—was increasing, although the Americans at that time were in Vietnam only in the role of advisers. Army reconnaissance planes had been increasingly subjected to ground fire.

Daily I heard talk, some of it not meant for my ears, that the war was drawing closer to us. Nhatrang, unlike many other provincial capitals, had not yet been subjected to Vietcong terror techniques, which commonly included the planting of plastic bombs and the assassination or kidnapping of government officials, minor functionaries and policemen. No one could be sure how long Nhatrang would remain free from trouble. The extension of the airfield to accommodate military jets, the new Military Assistance Advisory Group installations, the increase in American military personnel might all serve as an incentive for sneak attacks. Outlying villages and towns in the province had already suffered night raids but none were yet controlled by the Vietcong.

But all of this was vague, full of rumor. The full impact of what Vietcong activity could really amount to came at the end of May.

We learned that the Vietcong had kidnapped Dr. Ardel Vietti and two of her aides, including the paxman, from the Banmethuot leprosarium. They had also taken medicines, instruments for amputations, bedding, bandages, and one of the Land-Rovers. It appeared to be a well-planned maneuver, indicating their dire need for medical skill and equipment. This, then, was the reason the leprosarium had been under surveillance.

I was stunned. Dr. Dick calmly tried to sort out the facts from the rumors. There was hope that the captives would not be harmed because their skills were too valuable to destroy by death. But no one knew what brutality might be used to force them to comply with the enemy's demands. The whole subject of Vietcong atrocities was fabricated out of rumors—some indicating unspeakable horrors, others grossly contradicting them. All were undoubtedly colored by the political sympathy of the source of information.

What this meant for us was the question in all of our minds. The Chan-Y-Vien was probably better equipped for general medical needs than the leprosarium. And our medical experience in Vietnam gave us a broader background in treating the sick and maimed than did the specialized training of those who had been kidnapped. But, as Dr. Dick pointed out, it was the isolation of the leprosarium that made Dr. Vietti and her colleagues so vulnerable.

The location of the Chan-Y-Vien would make us a poor target for the Vietcong. We were in a fairly well-traveled area. There were an orphanage and a Bible school on adjoining property. The Vietnamese academy for noncommissioned officers, the U.S. Army training center, and the new Eighth Field Hospital, on whose doctors we so frequently called, were not far away. So we went on performing the services we were here for while hearing rumors and listening to stories, but never being fully persuaded that we were in any real danger.

8

FROM THEN ON we heard weekly and sometimes daily reports of violence in other parts of South Vietnam. These incidents occurred particularly in the Mekong Delta area and the Camau peninsula in the southernmost part of the long, narrow country, but we were informed of episodes elsewhere as well.

The Vietcong was surely the most mysterious of fighting forces. Nobody knew when or how it would strike next. Every new incident seemed to come as a complete surprise. Rarely did South Vietnamese military or American advisory personal have advance intelligence regarding Vietcong raids, bombings, or ambushes. It was more likely that planted "mis-intelligence" was their only source of information.

Who are the Vietcong? The label, provided by the regime of South Vietnam's President Ngo Dinh Diem, is an abbreviation for "Vietnamese Communists," although not all

Vietcong are Communists. It was estimated in 1963 that the hard-core fighting guerrillas numbered about 25,000 strong and that there were between 60,000 and 80,000 irregulars. The South Vietnamese regular army and various local military guard units at that time had almost 400,000 men. The Vietcong was an extremely mobile "shadow" force, relying for its success on speed, secrecy, and surprise. Operating individually or in small raiding and ambush parties, they conducted what one American military advisor described as "a sleight-of-hand war that kept everybody guessing but themselves."

In addition to these highly trained guerrillas, there were untold numbers of active Vietcong supporters who served as spies and couriers, and who provided food, shelter and hiding places for men and weapons. These "agents" were said to be drawn from all classes of the South Vietnamese including, it was rumored, bureaucrats working for the government. There were rumors also that spying occurred on all levels of the Vietnamese Army, and the number of desertions to the Vietcong was growing alarmingly; more than the government was willing to admit.

In Nhatrang and the surrounding countryside, as in most every other city, town and hamlet, these volunteer spies reportedly operated almost totally unhampered by the government. Not even the threat of death—the South Vietnamese penalty for treason—could curb or eliminate their activities. Those who might have exposed their neighbors, business associates, friends or government officials didn't do so for fear of reprisals from the Vietcong.

From the beginning the Vietcong operation was supported by President Ho Chi Minh of North Vietnam. Ho, himself a trained and resourceful guerrilla (as the defeated French had good reason to know), foresaw that only unconventional warfare against the Republic of South Vietnam could quickly bring large areas under Communist control. He provided these activities with a "liberation" label—the National Liberation Front of South Vietnam, or NLF—and helped set up political and administrative arms of the fighting forces to win the loyalty and sympathy of South Vietnam. Although many of its members were Communists and the organization appeared to be controlled and directed by Communists, the membership included a wide spectrum of political opinion and represented several different political factions. Its main purpose was to establish front organizations in villages and hamlets and to spread propaganda aimed at instilling a feeling of nationalism among the Vietnamese peasantry who were, until now, neither concerned with nor aware of political matters. Traditionally, the Vietnamese feel personal loyalty only to their families, and political loyalty only to their native villages. For centuries the central government had served solely as tax collector, army recruiter, and policeman. The new political cadres undertook to make all South Vietnamese, both peasant and intelligentsia, aware of the benefits communism would bring them. North Vietnam, Communist China and Russia underwrote the Vietcong by supplying munitions, and North Vietnam provided military forces as well. Ho Chi Minh refused to allow foreign advisors into the NLF so fears of a return to foreign domination would not be aroused.

Vietcong activities were then concentrated in the villages. The strategy alternated between benevolence and terrorism. When adverse weather conditions in 1961 had caused rice crops to fall below normal in many places, the Vietcong took advantage of this crop failure by setting up its own system of distributing, to loyal supporters, rice confiscated from more productive districts and government relief shipments. From what I heard, wholesale executions were not common as a means of enforcing loyalty. But when there was outright resistance to demands for rice, money, recruits and intelligence, a victim was chosen to be shot or beheaded as an example to the rest. Farmers who refused to yield a part or all of their crop might be executed for "a crime against the people." Young men might be forcibly taken away to serve with the Vietcong. To force a recalcitrant village into cooperation, the village chieftain, policeman, or schoolteacher might be put to death on a trumped-up charge of spying for the Saigon government. The women, often left homeless with young children and old and infirm parents to care for, would try as best they could to feed what remained of their families. If all this didn't always result in complete allegiance, at least the Vietcong could be certain of grudging cooperation.

In addition, regardless of how intense hostilities became, most South Vietnamese did not completely regard the Vietcong as a revolutionary force. A tradition of tolerance for variant beliefs and a feeling of relationship even to dissident fellow countrymen contributed to a general reluctance to betray them.

It was reported to us in 1962 that half of South Vietnam's countryside was pretty much in the control of the Vietcong. By blasting arterial highways, bridges, and rail lines, the rebels had succeeded in isolating whole sections of the country, including Saigon and most of the provincial capital cities. Nhatrang, however, had so far escaped, probably because it was a resort and not a business center. Those roads and rail lines which remained operational were under constant surveillance, so that the Vietcong were always informed of movements of soldiers and military supplies. They were able to ambush strategic convoys, killing or capturing military personnel and civilians as well as capturing materiel. On the roads controlled by the Vietcong, travel was strictly regulated. Goods in transit between cities were subject to a tax; failure to pay tribute resulted in the confiscation of produce and merchandise. Private property was also subject to confiscation. And, of course, smuggled or stolen government shipments and relief supplies were always "welcomed."

On the part of the Diem government, the most ambitious effort to counter terrorism was to set up strategic hamlets. This was a pet project of Ngo Dinh Nhu, Diem's brother and most important advisor. It was hoped that these hamlets would offer protection to about 10 per cent of the population. A sprawling village was to be subdivided into several smaller fortified units, each virtually a miniature armed camp. If each of these was completely capable of defending itself, the guerrilla raids would be ineffective and the Vietcong would be deprived of the food for which they were dependent on the villagers. Young men were trained and armed, but their guns were outmoded. Multiple rows of American barbed wire were erected around the selected areas. A curfew was ordered from six in the evening until dawn. Guard towers were built so that lookouts could detect members of the Vietcong who might try to slip in behind villagers returning from the fields. But the biggest hindrance to the success of this idea was that it disrupted the traditional village structure. And in most cases, Vietcong members friendly with or related to residents of the hamlets managed to get themselves fenced inside and could later form a "welcoming committee" to the raiders.

It may have been that many of our hospital patients acted as spies in their home districts and perhaps were even actively engaged in fighting, but I never had reason to suspect anyone. Since a number of the women and children who came for treatment lived in captured areas, it was quite likely that many of their husbands and fathers were Vietcong guerrillas. The Chan-Y-Vien was open to all, regardless of political loyalty, and patients' political affiliations were never questioned.

For the men forced to fight in the war, either on the side of the South Vietnamese or with the Vietcong, circumstances were often extremely difficult. Most of those called up or kidnapped were poor peasants or workers, with dependent wives and young children, and neither the government nor the insurgents provided payments to dependents. There was no insurance payable in the event of a soldier's death, and the wounded did not receive pensions. On both sides, those drafted were in service for the duration of the war. Some of the men with the South Vietnamese army had been in action since 1954 and had not seen or heard from their families since then. Furloughs were granted infrequently and, since the peasants were rarely able to read or write, there was virtually no communication between them. Word of a death sometimes took months to reach the soldier's family. On the other hand, wealthy and middle-class Vietnamese usually became regular or noncommissioned officers. I heard that the officers had recruits to carry their gear, do their cooking, set up their tents, string their hammocks, wash laundry, and in general make life as comfortable as possible.

One amenity available to even the poorest native soldier of both camps was the "bamboo telegraph." This time-honored Asian method of sending messages, remarkable for both its speed and accuracy, has been used for centuries where villages are usually miles apart and few people can read or write. It operates by passing along orally the name of the person to whom the message is going, his address, and the message itself. The information is given to a relative or someone from one's own village who is going in the direction of the recipient. There is always a great deal of coming and going between villages. It is not unusual for the messenger, whose destination may only take him part of the way toward the recipient, to deliver the message to another courier who will complete all or part of the journey. A message may be relayed through a number of people, and no gift or payment of any kind is made for this service.

It is assumed that at some time the favor will be reciprocated. In an emergency, a foreigner can usually find a native to send a message on its way.

At the Chan-Y-Vien we had frequent opportunity to admire the efficiency of the bamboo telegraph. Often I would say to a patient in the evening, "All right, you can go home tomorrow. Have someone come for you." And in the morning a member of the patient's family would appear, almost as if by magic.

It was remarkable that in this strife-torn country, subjected to foreign intrusion for so long, we felt absolutely no resentment toward us as aliens. The people seemed to go out of their way to try to include us in the happy events of their lives, and at one time I had so many invitations to teas and parties and weddings and dinners that I was only able to accept a fraction of them. It was therefore surprising to all of us when there was a misunderstanding of major proportions that involved the staff of the Chan-Y-Vien just before Dr. Dick's term of service was to expire.

Pastor Tin, who was chairman of the board of directors of our hospital, had asked Dr. Dick to provide medical examinations for a group of Vietnamese ministers who were in

Nhatrang for a convention. The doctor set aside two evenings for this. The patients were asked to pay the established clinic fee—it was an extremely modest ten piasters, or about twelve cents—but, apparently being used to receiving various services gratis because of their position, the clergymen refused. Rather than make an issue of it, we decided to waive the fee. The examinations proceeded without further incident until one patient demanded that it be repeated because he felt it hadn't been thorough. Dr. Dick, anticipating that all of them would demand recounts if he acceded, refused. The disgruntled patient then complained at length to Pastor Tin, who offered no defense of the staff. Dr. Dick, who had spent so much time at the Chan-Y-Vien, was particularly disturbed by the apparent lack of appreciation shown by Pastor Tin.

It happened that the next afternoon I was checking the clinic record books. The Vietnamese aides were supposed to keep the accounts of the clinic fee of ten piasters for the first visit, five for each succeeding visit. And when I added up the day's small receipts, there was a discrepancy. I asked Mimmie about it. She got very upset and immediately went home.

When she did not come to work the next day, we concluded that it was because of the disagreement with her father, Pastor Tin. Dr. Dick was still angry, and because we were now without an interpreter he decided to suspend clinic.

After a few days Pastor Tin came in to see Dr. Dick. "Marva accused my daughter of stealing," he announced. "Mimmie will not be working with you anymore."

When Dr. Dick reported this to me I felt terrible. Of course I had not accused her of stealing. I went to see Mimmie and explained to her that I was only trying to balance the books.

I realized from this episode that the misunderstanding between us grew out of our different ways of relating incidents and expressing ourselves. I resolved to be more careful and to try to anticipate what might prove offensive, thereby eliminating possible insults or even ruffled feelings.

After our talk, Mimmie decided to come back to us and clinic was resumed. The hospital routine was back to normal.

9

BA-MUOI, OUR COOK, and I had become good friends. And so she invited me to come to dinner on her day off, which was the following Sunday. I was particularly pleased at this invitation because, although it would not be my first visit to a Vietnamese home, it would be my first Vietnamese home-cooked meal.

Her home, which was within walking distance of the Chan-Y-Vien, was well furnished by Vietnamese standards. Her husband was a baker whose income permitted him some extra comforts. The house was of the traditional yellow stucco with a red tile roof. The floor of the two-room structure was of bright tile. There were colorful plastic flowers in vases and lacquered pictures on the walls. There were fluorescent lights, which I saw in many homes in Nhatrang, as opposed to the kerosene lamps which were common in houses in the countryside. Lovely orange, lime, papaya, jackfruit, coconut, and banana trees grew in front of Ba-muoi's house.

There were four of us that afternoon. In addition to Ba-muoi, her husband and myself, there was the wife of a pastor, a gracious woman who spoke English fairly well, whose husband was away for the day.

We sat down to one of the most sumptuous meals I have ever eaten. Until now I had regarded Ba-muoi as a perfunctory cook. The meals she prepared for us usually consisted of what she thought American food should be, and that was mostly overcooked. Squash, eggplant, or any other vegetable would be boiled until it was quite dry and tasteless. Her menus were predictable and dull, only occasionally enlivened by a Vietnamese dish. We could tell what day of the week it was from the dinner Ba-muoi served. But she proved to be truly proficient in her native cuisine and prepared a memorable meal. Although I can uncomplainingly eat poor cooking, I thoroughly enjoy good food, and Ba-muoi's dinner that Sunday was delicious.

We had chicken stuffed with transparent noodles, rice, and lotus buds; green squash, onions, and succulent chunks of beef prepared in a delectable sauce; a salad of green beans, cabbage, and chicken served over rice and topped with chopped peanuts; crisply fried pork surrounded by subtle sauces for dunking; and, at the end of the meal, a delicate clear soup, followed by tea.

But despite the fact that another guest spoke some English and that I had learned some Vietnamese, conversation during dinner was awkward. I didn't know what to say that would be of interest to them and they didn't know what would entertain me.

After dinner I was taken on a tour of the bakery. It occupied one large room of a long building behind Ba-muoi's house. There were three other rooms in this second structure. Two rooms were rented out and the third was occupied by Ba-muoi's son, daughter-in-law, and three grandchildren. In the baking room I saw wooden troughs used for mixing and shaping the long loaves of French style bread. Twenty or thirty loaves could bake at a time in the two brick ovens. And the smell of yeast, of bread rising, and loaves baking was just wonderful.

It was a pleasant interlude in a busy schedule, and I returned to the Chan-Y-Vien laden with fruits and flowers from my hostess, refreshed and ready for the week ahead.

Dr. Dick's three-year term of service was over. Before his departure a number of parties were held in his honor. It is a very old tradition in Vietnam to make the weeks before a person is to leave a time of great festivities. The largest and most elegant of the parties was arranged by the same group of ministers who had precipitated a quarrel with the doctor a month before. The passage of time had restored a friendly relationship, and the occasion provided an opportunity to prove that no remnant of unpleasantness remained.

The day of the Dicks' departure was very hot, but people from the villages around the Chan-Y-Vien came to the airport to see the doctor and his family leave, bringing with them all sorts of last-minute gifts. The most popular goodbye presents were huge lacquered pictures of romantic local scenes—I remember several almost identical views of great big seagulls hovering over a small boat. Since the Dicks obviously couldn't take all of them—some were quite bulky—into the plane, I was left with the problem of disposing of the extras without hurting anybody's feelings. Probably those lacquered pictures have remained in the Chan-Y-Vien's storeroom to this day.

Amid much cordial chatter from the crowd of well-wishers, the five members of the Dick family boarded the plane.

Dr. Dick's replacement, Dr. Yoder, was due to arrive in three weeks. Until then I would be on my own. The Lichtis were to stay with me at the bungalow in the meantime, but the brunt of the hospital work would, of course, be on my shoulders.

Those three weeks seemed to fly. Elda Lichti had come from Saigon prepared to redecorate the bungalow, which was desperately in need of a paint job, among other things. I had hoped to be able to help her, but there wasn't a minute to spare. While she and Anh Ba, the laundryman, turned the house from gray to refreshing blues, yellows and greens, I delivered five babies. While cupboards were stained and varnished, I examined over three hundred people in clinic. While new curtains were sewn and hung, I assisted the Army doctors at half a dozen operations, one of them an extremely successful procedure on the fisherman, Nam.

During this time we held our first dental clinic, courtesy of the U.S. Army. Days before, word went out through the bamboo telegraph that anyone with a toothache should come to the hospital on a specified day. By dawn of that day more than a hundred people were already assembled. A few hours later an Army truck arrived, containing a detail of dental corpsmen, two dental chairs, and all the equipment that would be needed. Two Army dentists followed in a jeep. Badly infected gums were treated and, in some cases, surgery was done. While they worked, the dentists explained what they were doing and had me assist at simple things. It was one of the most efficient maneuvers I had ever seen, and even included the activities of a cleanup squad at the end.

On a different occasion still another doctor came up specifically to teach me how to do blood counts and urinalyses —tests normally done by a laboratory technician. The Army medical staff's interest in teaching me what they could was an effort to make Chan-Y-Vien as self-sufficient as possible. Whatever training they could give me would, in the long run, make things much easier for them as well as me, since I would not have to call on them for these services.

One case that was very much on my mind during those weeks was that of Phi. He had appeared with his mother at clinic one morning, about two weeks before Dr. Dick left. He was about eight years old, dressed in tattered black clothes, and was so small and thin, with such enormous and beautiful eyes that I fell in love with him. The poor thing hopped about like a little bunny because one leg was bent back at a 45-degree angle. He had obviously had tuberculosis of the bone surfaces of the knee joint, and the resulting scar tissue had caused contracture of the muscles and tendons in his knee. He hadn't walked normally in over a year. Phi and his mother had come all the way from a village near Tuy Hoa, 50 miles to the north. Extensive orthopedic surgery and postoperative care would be needed to correct little Phi's deformity, and Dr. Dick was unable to take care of him at that time. He sent the child and mother back to their village, telling them we would let them know when an operation could be scheduled.

Dr. Dick left before he could attend to it, but I couldn't get the image of the small black-clad figure out of mind. I spoke of Phi to Dr. Walton, the orthopedic surgeon at the Army's Eighth Field Hospital, and he gave me hope that an operation could help the boy. I had been going to drive up to Phi's village, but part of the road was in Vietcong hands and it wasn't safe.

Dr. Walton decided to run up to Tuy Hoa himself in a helicopter to look for the boy. He took with him Dr. Tu, a surgeon at the Vietnamese Army hospital. They went in two small paramedic choppers, and buzzed me at the Chan-Y-Vien before they left. I wished I could go too; I had never been in a helicopter before and wanted to try it, and I was anxious to find little Phi.

They had some trouble locating the boy, but finally found him. A few hours later the pair of choppers hovered over the beach for a while to get my attention. They also attracted the attention of the children in the National Protesant Church orphanage just down the road from the Chan-Y-Vien, and all of them came running out to watch. Then the helicopters landed right in my front yard, and out stepped Phi, his mother, and a suckling baby.

After I settled the mother and baby in the ward, I put Phi under the shower and dressed him in clean clothing. Then I prepared him for what would be the first of many operations to straighten his leg. He came through the operation well and began the long process of recuperation. His mother was a Christian. She had several other children at home with relatives. His father had recently been killed by the Vietcong. She stayed for a few days, then came to me and said, "I'll just leave him here with you and God." And she departed, to somehow make her way back to her village.

At the end of July the Yoders arrived. I had met Dr. Carl and his wife Phyllis in the beginning of February, just before I left the States, at an orientation meeting provided by the M.C.C. for personnel about to serve abroad. They were an attractive couple, about my own age, then living in Lancaster, Pennsylvania, in an apartment just across the street from the Lancaster General Hospital. I liked them immediately and looked forward to working with them. I corresponded with them from time to time after I reached Vietnam, preparing them for what they would see when they came, answering their questions about what kind of medical problems we had, and about what to bring. Phyllis had asked if we could use a sewing machine. My answer was no, since we had one, although it was an old treadle model. She was also a nurse who would second me at the hospital in addition to taking care of the house.

I was delighted to greet the Yoders and show them around the Chan-Y-Vien.

One of the things I had written them about was the high incidence of problems requiring eye surgery. Dr. Yoder did special work in this area during his last months at Lancaster and, although he was not specifically trained as an eye surgeon, he came prepared to operate on entropions, cataracts, and a variety of other conditions.

Shortly after the Yoders arrived, we received a petition for medical help from Phi's village. His mother had told her neighbors what we were doing for the boy, and the village, filled with refugees who had defied the Vietcong, had large numbers of sick and injured who wanted us to help them.

Dr. Walton decided to organize a mobile medical clinic for an expedition to the area and asked Dr. Yoder if I could go along as nurse-interpreter. He agreed and offered his own and his wife's services as well. In addition there were three Army nurses. With a large supply of medical equipment in tow, we all set out in two helicopters.

An enormous crowd—it seemed like the whole village—was waiting for us. They had torn down some huts to make a landing pad and built a bamboo and palm leaf building of three rooms for our use. We worked from early in the morning until late in the afternoon, stopping only briefly for lunch and we were often forced to press the helicopter crews into assisting us. Records kept by the Army staff showed that altogether over 650 patients were examined and treated, over 200 teeth were extracted, more than 12,000 vitamin pills were distributed, and over 200 penicillin injections were administered. One impromptu operation took place, an amputation of the stump of a finger that had already been cut off. And those patients who the doctors felt needed more extensive surgical or medical treatment were told to come to the Chan-Y-Vien within the next few weeks. They were given notes to bring with them to identify them and their ailments.

For the Yoders this was an intensive introduction to what they were to find in Vietnam in the following months. For all of us it was an enriching experience, our first in full collaboration with the military on a common humanitarian project.

During the next few weeks I found myself increasingly tired and irritable. We were all working very hard since the numbers of patients visiting the clinic and in the ward had soared. But I felt that it was more than physical fatigue. Despite all the activity, I felt restless. Perhaps it was just a normal depression, a letdown feeling after the intoxicating effect of my first few months in Vietnam. Sometimes I just longed to go off for a day all by myself—to go sailing perhaps, surrounded only by the serenity of ocean and sky.

One thing that could be counted on to cheer me up was little Phi, with his large black eyes fringed with thick long lashes, his friendly smile, and his child's chatter. I would take him down to the beach several times a week, to exercise his leg in the ocean.

Dr. Walton was fond of the child, too, and came over

whenever he could to see how he was getting on. He was so interested in Phi that I would find myself thinking of him as "Dr. Walton's little boy." One day the three of us went into Nhatrang to get Phi some new clothes. The undersized Vietnamese lad hopped along on crutches between the two tall Americans having the time of his young life.

He stayed at the hospital for quite a while. He was a docile child—most Vietnamese children are well behaved—and never got into mischief. Because he was alone and so small and had been there for so long, he never had any one particular bed; we kept shifting him around like a little mascot.

In the evening if I finished my work early it was my custom to spend some time talking with the ward patients. I would sit at the foot of a bed and make conversation. At first I would ask them about themselves, but after a while they began to feel more at ease and they would ask me questions. They were very curious about America. So many things I took for granted were virtually indescribable to someone who had never experienced them. They would ask how cold it became in winter, and what snow tasted like. They wanted to know why the buildings grow high in the sky and whether people didn't get terribly tired climbing to the top. At some point I mentioned the subway, and this was totally inconceivable to them. But even more than the physical aspects of America they wanted to know about our way of life. Why didn't children perform useful work? It was then that I realized how much easier it is to describe how elevators work, what snow looks and feels like, and how enormous tunnels are constructed under a city for mass transportation than to explain the differences in our social practices.

Early one evening when I sat down at the foot of Phi's bed, he said he was still hungry. Perhaps he really was, or perhaps, like little children everywhere, he wanted extra attention. I had earlier given him a few piasters to buy his food from the vendors, as I did every day, since there was no one to cook for him after his mother left. Sometimes the other patients would share their meals with him. But this evening he insisted that he was hungry. I decided that the lonely child was certainly entitled to some extra fussing over, and I told him to wait while I found something for him to eat.

In a cupboard I discovered some Vietnamese goodies left by another patient, and I brought them back to the little fellow. He smiled his thanks as he began to eat. But he wouldn't let me leave him. So I tucked him in and told him that instead of going back to my own room at the bungalow, I would spend the night near him on the next bed. Apparently this was just what he needed, for he relaxed and in a few moments fell asleep.

10

CHILDREN WERE a common sight in the ward at the Chan-Y-Vien. We had many of them, of all ages, and the most frequent condition for which they were hospitalized was tuberculosis. It was frustrating to realize that the most significant factor contributing to the high incidence of this disease was inadequate nutrition. Medication was capable of effecting a cure over a period of time. But the fact that the disease was so prevalent and that an undernourished child was destined to grow into a constitutionally weakened adult made its recurrence almost inevitable.

Most of the children were brought to us by their mothers or grandmothers. I came to believe that it was really the old ladies who were running Vietnam, the grannies, constantly chewing betel nut, who took care of their children and children's children, staying with them in the ward if necessary, each bringing food and comfort to a cooped-up youngster.

But one of my favorite child patients appeared one day all

by himself. He was about ten years old, a little small for his age, with a shock of thick black hair. His name, he said, was Hai; and like so many of the others, he had tuberculosis.

After he had been with us for a few days he felt well enough to respond to my overtures of friendship. "Co," he said, "I will tell you about Hai." *Co-Y-Ta*, the patients called me; it means "Miss Nurse." Hai always referred to himself in the third person.

He had been born, he told me, in a rural hamlet in the hills some 300 miles northwest of Nhatrang. His full name was Nguyen-Hai. Hai is the number two in Vietnamese. He explained that it meant he was the firstborn child of his parents. To call a child by the number one would be to call special attention to him, to point him out to the devil. So the first child is called "Two" to fool the devil, to turn his attention elsewhere.

When Hai was two years old his father was drafted into the army. His mother, from his description very young and very beautiful, was left on her own to feed and support herself and her child. Her family had left the area to settle not far from Nhatrang shortly after she married and so she had no relations nearby to help her. The village in which they lived was poor and there was no help from neighbors.

For several years nothing was heard from Hai's father. And then, one day, they received word that he had been killed in a skirmish. His mother, destitute and unhappy, agreed to marry one of the village elders, a harsh and rigid widower who regarded Hai as a spoiled troublemaker. For some reason the marriage wasn't to take place for a year. But the husband-to-be took it upon himself to train and discipline the little boy. This involved long hours of work far too difficult for such a youngster and, more often than not, was rewarded with beatings.

Shortly before the wedding was to occur, Hai's father returned to the village. He had deserted from the South Vietnamese Army and it had taken him many months, traveling as a fugitive by night, to reach his home. When he arrived he was emaciated, sick, and unable to work. Since Hai's mother had to devote all her time to nursing him, Hai was hired out to the widower he had come to despise.

When Hai's father was well enough to travel, the family decided to move to another village where there was less chance of being discovered by government officials. They were in their new home just a short time when Vietcong raids began. During the first raid their home was destroyed and their meager crops burned. During the second raid Hai's father was taken away by the Vietcong and was never heard from again. During the third raid Hai's mother was killed by a stray bullet.

The remaining villagers decided it would be best if Hai was sent to his mother's family near Nhatrang. A few weeks later the elders learned that a man and wife from a nearby village were going there and would consent to take Hai with them. Walking part of the distance and hitching rides for the rest of the journey, Hai and his escorts slowly made their way down to the sea.

Finally he arrived in the fishing village of his relatives to find his aunt with her husband and three children still there. She reluctantly took him in. To earn his keep Hai became one of the village watchmen, staying up night after night to alert the community in the event of a raid. He received virtually no attention from the impoverished remnant of his family. When he became sick, one of his older cousins took him part of the way to the Chan-Y-Vien and pointed out the direction. That was why he had come on foot, alone.

I had heard so many stories like Hai's that I knew everything he told me was true. His matter-of-fact acceptance of his life made my own impulse to pity him naïve. Tears in Vietnam were useless.

When Hai was well I would have to find a place for him, a home where he would be welcomed during the few years of childhood that were left him.

And so Hai and I became "buddies." He was an ingratiating child and tried to help me whenever he could. He would run errands for me and amuse the children who came to clinic while I worked with their parents. I recognized, of course, that he was trying to make himself indispensable in the hope that he could remain at the hospital indefinitely. And I tried to reassure him that I would look after him, that I would try to find a place for him when he was well.

At that time my parents were particularly worried about my safety. I gathered from their letters that South Vietnam was constantly in the American headlines, with emphasis being placed on Vietcong terrorism. And they had, of course, learned of the kidnapping from the leprosarium. There was still no word of the three staff members.

Our only sources of information, aside from rumor, about what was really happening were nightly news broadcasts over shortwave radio and back issues of newspapers and magazines from home. We were completely uninformed about day-to-day developments away from the hospital.

The letters I wrote home usually avoided mention of the war and concentrated on activities at the Chan-Y-Vien. I constantly reassured my family that there was no military activity around Nhatrang, but at the same time they were reading about the increased number of American troops being sent into the area. I kept stressing the tremendous satisfaction I was receiving from my work. I told them, truthfully, that the Vietcong was something we really knew almost nothing about from firsthand experience.

Occasionally we would joke about the situation. One time

a patient who had been hospitalized with a severely infected finger and who had a wife and five children waiting at home, decided, against our advice, to leave. "But," I remonstrated, "you'll lose the use of your finger if you go home now; stay a few more days."

He appeared to have consented, but when I went into the ward next morning I discovered that he had left during the night. I told Dr. Yoder and Phyllis, and we decided, "Well, he must be an essential member of the Vietcong."

But mostly we thought of the Vietcong only in terms of the hardships this shadowy fighting force imposed on our patients. A lot of them came from villages that were occupied, or had to travel through occupied territory to reach the Chan-Y-Vien. A patient would be told to return for further medication in a month. But at that time someone else would appear with a message saying "I can't get out. Please give my medicine to my friend."

One father walked for two nights through jungles, carrying his seventeen-year-old daughter. He had an eye infection, and the pitifully frail girl was suffering from a rare pancreatic disease. We were able to take care of the man's eye, but the daughter, his only child, died. The father couldn't possibly take her body surreptitiously all that distance back home.

"What will I do?" he asked us sadly. "I can't take her home. And I have no money to bury her."

In the meantime the man's wife had come down. We were able to arrange for burial at the potter's field maintained by the Province Hospital. For a few hundred piasters, which the Chan-Y-Vien paid, the Province Hospital provided a box and winding sheets. The body was placed in the coffin, which was put on a truck, with a candle at the head and feet, and this most pathetic of funeral processions was on its way.

So we were always aware of the Vietcong's ghostly presence, although we were never personally threatened. We knew it was there, in an indefinite area usually about fifteen miles away, although sometimes it was a closer specter.

In August my father wrote to ask me if I would attend the Pan-Pacific Rehabilitation Conference in his place; it was to be held in Manila in November. He explained that he was unable to be there to represent the American Leprosy Missions. He knew of my interest in the field of rehabilitation and he was glad to be able to offer me a pleasant change of pace. I looked forward to meeting the other participants in the conference, some of whom I knew from India, others of whom were well known in this field.

Because of my work with Dr. Walton's mobile medical clinic, I was able to fly to Manila gratis, courtesy of the U.S. government, on a C-123 medical evacuation plane. I was listed as a medical attendant and my patient was an army captain. Although the plane had several serious litter cases, my own patient's disability was limited to an arm in a sling. He was therefore more my attendant than I his and I thoroughly relaxed and enjoyed the flight. My first night in Manila was spent at the hospital at Clark Air Force Base, and in the morning I took a bus to the downtown auditorium where for the next few days I would be thoroughly engrossed in discussions of the physical, emotional, and psychological aspects of rehabilitation.

As the summer moved into fall the hospital became increasingly busy. We were receiving many more than the usual number of clinic patients and emergency cases.

One evening, a *xich-lo* came up to the verandah of the Chan-Y-Vien and a woman carrying a child got out. Since it was well after clinic hours we knew that only an emergency would have brought them. Dr. Yoder and I took them directly into his office.

I recognized her as a former clinic patient. Her husband, a wounded soldier, was confined to the military hospital in Nhatrang and she lived about a mile from the hospital.

Both mother and child had been bitten by a poisonous snake, a kind of elapidae. The child had the characteristic double fang marks on his foot; the mother's marks were on her upper thigh. They had most likely been bitten when they went outdoors to relieve themselves; the mother receiving the first bite and the child the second, less potent one.

Dr. Yoder immediately administered anti-elapidae serum to mother and son. Then he slashed the mother's wound and applied a suction pump in the hope of drawing off enough venom with the blood to prevent a lethal amount from entering the circulatory system. I tied a tourniquet below the child's knee to slow his blood circulation and then attached a suction pump to the incision I made on his foot.

By midnight the boy was past the crisis. Both the location and severity of his wound were less dangerous than that of his mother. But the woman had lapsed into unconsciousness and there was little hope of her emerging from the coma.

Dr. Yoder had been at work since before dawn that day and I urged him to rest while I watched over the patients. There was little more we could do for them except wait. Within an hour the young mother died. I covered her with a blanket and carried the sleeping child into the ward. I checked his respiration and found it satisfactory. Hai had heard me come in and I asked him to watch over the child. I knew it would be several hours before I got back.

100

Next I went into the doctor's office to clean up. Then I put the woman's body on a litter and into the Land-Rover. I would take her home to her relatives. Handling the dead was, of course, part of my training. I don't know if I'm any more inured to it than anybody else. But by then I had become quite accustomed to taking a dead patient home when there was no way for a relative to come for the body.

It was an eerie night, windy and rainy, and I did not look forward to my ride. As I got into the truck to drive off, I heard a rustling noise coming from the shadows in the direction of the hospital. I turned, startled, but was reassured when I recognized Anh Tin, one of our most helpful aides. He had heard me working late and, coming from his quarters to help, had seen me putting the body into the truck. Surmising my destination, he said, "I will go with you, to help you find your way in the dark." At any other time I would have told him not to bother, but now I was glad of his company.

Driving past the tumbledown shacks along the road and hearing the wind whistle through them, you felt as if you yourself were already drawn into the tomb. The atmosphere of the night really affected me—that, and my sad burden. I thought of the helplessness of so many of these people, forced out of their traditional homes. I reflected on the sense of complete aloneness that death always brings to mourners. I wondered at the reception I would receive from the dead woman's family; at least I could tell them that the child would survive.

Anh Tin's presence was a comfort during that depressing ride. It was so dark that I could barely make out the landmarks by which I usually found my way. Anh Tin kept his eye peeled for the large mango tree that was just beyond the turn-off. As I was about to pass it, he spied it and tugged my arm to turn the wheel.

A light indicated the house we were looking for. We slowed down. An elderly woman emerged from the entrance and approached us. We stopped. "You have brought my daughter to me," she said, a statement of fact, not a question. I nodded, but it wasn't necessary. In some way she knew that her daughter had died. I was astonished to find that all the funeral preparations had already been arranged.

Anh Tin and I expressed our condolences in the appropriate Vietnamese manner while two neighbors went to the rear of the truck and removed the body. The woman covered her face with her hands. We followed her into the small house. Outside the wind was still blowing and a cold rain was falling, but the house was warm and fragrant from the candles and incense that were burning.

In the flickering light I could make out the objects in the room. There was a crude wooden coffin lined with sawdust. I was startled to see it there; less than four hours had passed since the mother and child had come to the hospital. The old woman obviously had believed, with characteristic Vietnamese fatalism, that her daughter would not survive the night.

While the body was transferred to the coffin, the other mourners—neighbors—came in. They formed a semi-circle around the coffin and began chanting. Anh Tin later explained to me that they were beseeching the young mother's ancestors to treat her kindly and would continue these supplications until the sun came up. Members of the family wept silently, as the wailing of the wind permeated the house. My eyes had begun to burn from the incense. Unnoticed by the mourners, Anh Tin and I left. We still had a rainy drive through the dark night before us.

11

Two DAYS BEFORE Christmas we held services for the staff
and patients at the Chan-Y-Vien with the prayers and sermon delivered in Vietnamese. Afterward the Yoders held
an informal party in the bungalow. Each member of the staff
was given a gift—a quilt made by a Mennonite farm wife
in Pennsylvania. Although it was not quite like a traditional
family gathering, it had some of the flavor of Christmas at
home and I felt less homesick than I thought I would.

The Yoders left the next day for Hue, where they would
be spending Christmas week with Phyllis' parents. Her father, head of the English department at Goshen College, a
Mennonite school in Indiana, was spending his sabbatical
year teaching American and English literature at the University of Hue. Dr. Samuel Yoder (Phyllis' maiden name was
the same as her married name) and his wife were in Vietnam on a Smith-Mundt grant.

I would therefore be in charge of the hospital for a few days. Hopefully, the patient load would be light. Our only serious case when the Yoders left was the girl we called "Sleeping Beauty"—a tiny three-year-old who had been almost constantly in a coma for the two weeks she was with us. Suffering from tubercular meningitis, she had been brought from Dalat by her parents, an attractive young couple, both of whom were half Chinese. The girl was their only child. Everything possible was being done to save her, but she had so far failed to respond to the treatment, which consisted of relatively massive oral doses of isoniazid and streptomycin injections. It seemed that only a miracle would bring her out of the deepening coma. I prayed for this.

On Christmas Eve things were quiet at the hospital and, since Anh Tin was on duty, I was able to take part in the service at the Army chapel. Anh Tin had become the most skilled of our Vietnamese aides. He had started at the Chan-Y-Vien as a sweeper, but because he was bright, literate and anxious to help he had been given increased responsibilities. We could call on him at any time and he always justified our confidence in him.

So now, when the chaplain invited me to attend services and play the organ, I was happy to oblige. The service was conducted early in the evening instead of at midnight because of curfew restrictions. And every member of that congregation—far from home and on duty in a strange country —was feeling alone and lonely.

When I left the chapel after the service, accompanied by the chaplain and a sergeant who was to drive the jeep, I was reminded that our trip back to the hospital was considered dangerous because it was outside the city limits. The canvas top of the jeep had been removed so that we could make a hasty exit in the event of an attack. But the trip through the quiet night was, as always, uneventful.

On Christmas day the clinic was closed. The Army chaplain had planned to fly to four outlying U.S. bases to conduct services. I was invited to go along to play the organ. We would take off at about 6 o'clock in the morning and be back in the early afternoon. I left two workers on duty in our hospital ward. The condition of the unconscious "Sleeping Beauty" had neither improved nor worsened. Her mother was with her constantly—watching, waiting, and hoping that the little one would wake and stir.

As per schedule the chaplain picked me up only minutes after I had checked all the ward patients and given the workers their final instructions. At the airfield, the pilot and copilot of a single-engine Otter awaited us. Already aboard the small plane was a portable organ. It was a small pump organ, especially built for the field, and weighed only about 35 pounds. From their remarks, the crew regarded the day's tour with a lady organist as something of a lark. The small, slow plane was eventually airborne and we set out on a northern course along the coast to a small base at Tuy Hoa.

Half an hour later, we lost altitude, buzzed the base, and landed on a short strip close by the sea. Our welcoming committee was the disinterested driver of a jeep. He offered no assistance in getting the organ out of the Otter, so we handled our own gear. We paused first at the mess hall for coffee with the commanding officer and members of his staff. Later, walking along a covered portico to the game room where the service would be held, I noticed a dozen Vietnamese squatting in the open. They were guarded by an armed Vietnamese soldier. The American military assistance officer escorting us explained that it was a group of captured

Vietcong suspects who would shortly be marched off to begin a day's work on the roads, Christmas or no Christmas.

Less than two dozen Americans attended the Episcopal service. They sang the Christmas hymns of rejoicing much as schoolboys would and sat through the chaplain's brief sermon with blank faces. They were loneliness personified.

Our next stop was at Pleiku, a much larger and better equipped installation. After the service we were invited to join the base for its traditional Christmas dinner—turkey, stuffing, cranberry sauce and all the trimmings flown in frozen from the States. After we left we flew inland to yet another base at Kontum. But we were now well behind schedule, and our visit had been written off. The game room that had been set aside for the service was empty. The bar on the base, however, was doing a lively business. The chaplain decided it would be more tactful for us to leave than to try rounding up a congregation of happily tipsy soldiers. Realizing that a similar after-dinner situation would greet us at our next stop, he cancelled our visit to the fourth base. So we returned to Nhatrang.

New Year's Eve was not a happy time for either the Yoders or myself. They had returned from Hue during the week to find that a number of new and seriously ill patients had been admitted to the ward, as well as a heavy influx of outpatients to the daily clinics. On top of these demands, it had become apparent that the life of the little girl we called "Sleeping Beauty" could not be saved. On New Year's Eve the mother, who was in constant attendance at the child's bedside, asked me to drive into town and send a wire to the father in Dalat, telling him to return to the hospital.

Telegrams were sent through the post office, and cost the equivalent of between ten and twenty cents. They were usually not delivered in person, but instead a note would be placed in the recipient's mail box advising him to call at his local post office to receive the message.

As often as possible, when making quick trips into Nha-trang, I tried to turn them into outings for Hai and as many convalescent patients as could be crammed into the Land-Rover. This night the car was jammed to capacity with kids and nearly-well older patients. None of course knew that my mission was a sad one, and they all had a grand time. On the way back, I drove slowly past the brightly lighted shops so they could all take a good look. The shops were doing a brisk business in anticipation of Tet, the Vietnamese lunar New Year, which would occur in mid-January. We stopped at a sweet shop and I bought candy and cookies for the Land-Rover's passengers. At least they would have a happy evening.

Back at the hospital, they went quietly to bed. I relieved Phyllis and stayed through the night with the mother beside the still form of the child, who died the next morning just before the father arrived.

By the second week of January, the number of outpatients had dwindled to less than eighty a day. The lunar New Year was nearing and required extensive preparations. Tet, a celebration in honor of ancestors, is the most important holiday in Vietnam and lasts three days. During that time no work is done, and every effort is made to spend the holiday with one's family. At the Chan-Y-Vien this meant that all of the patients who could would be allowed to go home and that the clinic wouldn't be operating, since it was doubtful that anybody would come.

Those patients who had to remain because they were too ill to travel, or too far from home, would stay at our newly acquired annex. We planned to take advantage of the lessened work load to give the hospital a much needed paint job. The annex was the nearby building that had been the home of Pastor Tin. He had been appointed professor at the Bible School up the hill and had been given a house there. So we now had additional quarters: two main rooms and several smaller ones to provide space for an overflow of patients and for guests.

To help Hai celebrate Tet, Phyllis and I took him to Nhatrang to buy a new wardrobe; it was customary for the Vietnamese to start their New Year wearing new clothing. We also bought him a Mai tree, as important during Tet as a fir tree is at Christmas in America.

It was the eve of Tet when the three of us went into town and every store and market stall was jammed with people doing their last-minute shopping. The streets and sidewalks were so crowded that we could barely get through. Little Hai, proudly holding one of my hands and one of Phyllis', was content to let us run interference for him while he looked with wide-eyed wonder at the splendors around him.

When we finished shopping, we stopped at the base of a hill that was topped by the ancient Cham Pagoda. The small building, set among ruins, is all that remains of a once imposing temple that looked down on the harbor. It is reached by steep steps well worn through the centuries by the feet of devout Buddhists. Brightly colored lanterns lit our way. At the stone paved terrace outside the pagoda, we removed our shoes and went quietly into the dim interior of the shrine. Hai left us standing near the door and went to kneel down with the other worshippers. In the gloom that was dank with age and misty from incense, we could barely make out the statue of Buddha at the altar. Tables laden with food offerings were in front of the Buddha. Pictures of Buddhist saints and revered abbots and priests were displayed on easels. The service, if it could be called that—people came and went at will to kneel and mumble prayers—was conducted by a priest garbed in gray who stood at one side of the altar. At intervals he would strike a flat, circular gong with a padded hammer. The dull, muted boom hung in the air for many seconds sounding like the voice of doom. The rise and fall of this eerie sound over the muffled prayers of the worshippers was quite awesome.

I watched Hai, kneeling with his hands pressed palm to palm before his lowered face. He was at this moment so different from the lively boy I knew. Like everyone around him, he was praying for the souls of his ancestors. This reverence is innate in all Vietnamese, even those who have professed Christianity.

The next day Hai's somber mood disappeared and in its place there was a gaiety I had rarely seen before. After breakfast I learned the reason. His Mai tree had bloomed on the first day of Tet, a very lucky omen for the Vietnamese. Later that day he told me that he knew the next year would be a good one for him. "You and me, Co," he said, "lucky-lucky until next Tet." There was an implication that after the next Tet our luck might change but I didn't ask him if that was what he meant.

The Yoders and I celebrated Tet by getting our painting program at the hospital into action. On the first of the festive days we had a "G.I. party." Several soldiers had volunteered to help us. They moved all the beds out of the ward into the yard, got the ward scrubbed down, painted the walls and window casements, and applied white enamel to the beds. If there's anything a man learns in the army, it's how to scrub and paint. These fellows, all young and in great spirits, went at their voluntary work with obvious enjoyment.

When the job was completed, it was decided to let the beds remain outside overnight to dry.

Early on the second morning of Tet, just when the Yoders and I were admiring the gleaming white beds out in our palm grove, a Lambretta puttered up. A man who literally looked like death itself was carried out by a friend. The friend told us quickly that the sick man, a fisherman from a village near Hue, had been "hit" by the "poisoned wind" during the night while at sea. Then the well man got back into the Lambretta and was driven off.

Almost every ailment was ascribed by the Vietnamese to poisonous winds, and patients would come in swathed in blankets to keep the wind away. We learned to go along with this figure of speech and, instead of saying "What are your symptoms?" we would ask "How did the wind hit you?"

But we didn't have to ask in this case. The patient was absolutely prostrate, and losing copious amounts of fluid by continuous diarrhea. We brought a stretcher as a temporary bed for the stricken man. While Dr. Yoder examined him, Phyllis and I, helped by Hai, took one of the beds from the yard back into the ward. Dr. Yoder came in and told us he was pretty sure the man had cholera. He suggested leaving the bed in the center of the empty room for now, so that we could easily get to the patient to give him the emergency treatment he required.

Dr. Yoder had never seen a cholera case before and was cautious about his diagnosis. But there had been rumors of such cases in both Hue and Saigon, which made it likely that the fisherman had brought the disease with him.

We sent Hai scurrying to find old newspapers, telling him to leave them in the clinic room and then to stay away from the hospital. The three of us had of course been innoculated against cholera before leaving the States, and we would be the only persons to have contact with our patient. We

110

weren't sure it was cholera, but we weren't taking any chances.

The rest of the day, Dr. Yoder observed the man closely and soon there was no question—he had cholera. When he came to us, the fisherman could not have been ill for more than a few hours. But his skin was already tight and drawn, and his eyes were sunk deep in their bony sockets. He already looked like a skeleton, so quickly had his body dehydrated from the rapid drain of fluids. For the next twenty-four hours Dr. Yoder kept two intravenous bottles going at the same time, trying desperately to stem the dehydration by giving at least as much fluid as was being lost. After that time the infection would abate and the patient probably would begin to retain fluid once more. At least 18 liters of solution must have entered the sick man's veins that day. In addition, supplementary bicarbonate solutions were administered orally by the glassful. We worked constantly to keep the patient's fluid intake at least equal to his emissions, which drained through the bare boards of the bed onto the pile of newspapers we had placed on the floor.

Every hour seemed a year—but we had the satisfaction of seeing the man still alive.

It was necessary to notify local health authorities that there was a highly contagious cholera patient at the Chan-Y-Vien. The fact that it was Tet and there was virtually no activity in Nhatrang made no difference. Leaving Phyllis and me at the man's bedside, Dr. Yoder went to tell the bad news to the chief medical officer at the Province Hospital. They returned together to the Chan-Y-Vien, and the Vietnamese doctor concurred with Dr. Yoder's diagnosis. Since we had no isolation facilities, it was decided to set up a tent outside the Province Hospital and transfer the patient there the following day.

Accordingly, at around ten the next morning, up drove the

Province Hospital ambulance. The attendants, wearing caps, gowns, masks, and rubber gloves, quickly put the patient in the ambulance and sped off. I promptly turned charwoman and thoroughly cleaned and disinfected the ward and the bed that had been occupied by the fisherman.

The end of this cholera case almost passes belief. That same afternoon, the patient received permission from the Province Hospital staff to return to his home. He was emaciated and extremely weak from his harrowing brush with death, but otherwise practically back to normal. We understood that he sailed at once for Hue. We were soon to discover that this feat was not unusual. Cholera is a severe and highly contagious bacterial infection but it lasts only a relatively short time. If its debilitating effect is immediately countered by the introduction of sufficient fluid, the body's own natural recuperative power succeeds in overcoming the infection. Death from cholera is actually caused by the complete and sudden dehydration that occurs if the victim does not receive adequate and prompt treatment.

12

I HAD BECOME ACQUAINTED with a woman named Kim Hoa some time after I arrived in Vietnam. At our first meeting I wasn't aware that she owned and operated, along with other members of her family, a beauty shop in Nhatrang, which I would later patronize occasionally.

The morning we met I was immediately struck by her appearance. She wore slim purple slacks and a short floral overblouse instead of the traditional *ao-dai*. What she was wearing was the equivalent of Western-style clothing. This young mother was bringing her pretty five-year-old daughter to the clinic. Both were shy, quiet, and sweet and their graciousness made a striking contrast to the less refined village women in the crowded clinic.

Trang, her daughter, had a flaccid right arm. Due to a birth injury the little girl was unable to exert muscular control over her arm and it hung limply by her side. Trang was admitted to the ward and examined by both Dr. Yoder and the Army orthopedic surgeon. They decided that muscle transplants just above her elbow would give her some movement and use of the arm. Tendons would be taken from the child's foot and used to lengthen the elbow muscle. As this required a series of operations over a period of time, Trang was with us for several weeks. During that time Kim Hoa, whom I later called Chi Hai, a less formal name meaning "Sister Two," became a good friend.

I learned that she was married to a young lieutenant in the Vietnamese Air Force. Trang, the oldest of her five children, was adopted. Trang had been found on the Nhatrang beach by a *xich-lo* driver only a few hours after she was born. It was assumed that she had been abandoned, rejected by her own parents because of the birth injury. The man took the infant to his home, but because he already had seven children he offered the baby to Kim Hoa and her husband. At that time they had been married for two years and still had no children. So she was their little girl, unaware of her origin or advent into this gracious home. She was loved dearly, and thoroughly pampered. The Vietnamese know how to pamper their small children. After Trang was discharged from the hospital, the Yoders and I were dinner guests of Kim Hoa and her family at their home, which adjoined the beauty parlor. We dined on asparagus and crab soup, shark fin rolled up in a lettuce leaf and dipped in *nuoc mam*, steamed white rice, and fried rice. The dessert was not ice cream but free trial hairdos for Phyllis and me, which were the first of many for both of us.

Kim Hoa was never critical of American military personnel in Nhatrang, although they were now apparent in substantial numbers. When I visited her shop, which was usually crowded with young girls getting elaborate upswept hairdos called "Saigon fashion," my appearance resulted in some looks and whispers. I knew the main reason was my blonde hair, so different in both color and texture from the thick, wavy dark hair of the Vietnamese. But conversations with Kim Hoa made me aware that I was the object of such scrutiny mainly because I was an American woman, a sight far more unusual than an American man.

Kim Hoa told me that many of the girls, even some from good families, were becoming involved with G.I.s. Many of them had received gifts—watches, rings, bracelets—along with promises of marriage from their American sweethearts. Kim Hoa repeatedly told them when they confided in her that these promised marriages would never take place. "In one year these men will go home and forget to write," she told me, repeating the warning she had so often given to the girls. But though many of those young women would believe her and knew this was so from previous experience of their own or of friends, they were not deterred from living for the benefits of the day. In the manner of many young people everywhere, they felt tomorrow would care for itself.

It was through Kim Hoa that I met her sister-in-law, Nga. Nga had spent nearly ten years in France, and when she returned worked as a bilingual secretary in Saigon. She also learned English. Nga heard about the hospital from Kim Hoa and came to Dr. Yoder asking him to do thyroid surgery. For years she had had a toxic thyroid, getting no relief from the French medicines she was given in Saigon. After several weeks of conservative therapy and medication, Dr. Yoder made arrangements for her to have surgery at the Province Hospital in Nhatrang. It would be done by an American surgeon. The Province Hospital was one of several in Vietnam that were now being partially staffed by civilian medical teams—doctors and nurses—provided by the United States Operations Mission (U.S.O.M.).

When Nga came to Nhatrang she brought with her a blond-haired boy who became the object of much curiosity. Nga explained quite casually that this was her son and that the father was an American G.I. who had left Vietnam when the child was only several months old. He had promised Nga that he would return in one year and marry her. Two years had now gone by and he had not returned. She had not even heard from him.

Nga's surgery was successful. It so happened that during the time she was recuperating, we lost Joe, the best interpreter our hospital ever had. Actually his name was Minh, but he wanted to be known as Joe. He was commandeered by the C.I.A. to work as an interpreter for them—as well as chief bar boy and best friend of the fliers of the Cockpit Club, one of the officers' clubs on base. We missed Joe pitifully, just as we had missed Mimmie when she had left us some time before, to get ready for her wedding.

But Nga, hearing of our need for an interpreter, offered her services and soon became an invaluable aid in the hectic struggle of each day's clinic. Nga also became one of my closest friends. Because of her fluency in English and her ability to anticipate what might be needed for a patient's care, it was possible to see and treat many more people in the daily clinics.

Nga lived in a house with another family, in a small room of her own close by the sea. Often we would talk, sharing ideas, hopes and dreams as we walked under the palm trees with the sounds of the pounding sea in the background. During this time her little boy, Jimmie, was living with her mother in Saigon.

Besides her job as interpreter with our hospital, Nga had a

part-time position as cashier in one of the town's snack bars, owned and run by an Indian. The place was a favorite haunt of American boys looking for steak sandwiches and a beer. There, one night, Nga met Charles, a carefree young G.I. As their friendship grew, she confided, Charles asked her to marry him. She had fears and doubts, however, because of her previous unhappy experience. But about two months before the end of Charles' tour in Vietnam, Nga discovered that she was pregnant. Charles persuaded her to apply for the necessary papers from both the U.S. Army and the Vietnamese government so that she could marry and go abroad. The process is long and difficult and the outcome is never certain. Then Charles had to leave. He promised to do everything in his power to expedite matters when he got to the States. Nga continued to work with us until she could no longer hide the secret of her pregnancy. She knew she must soon leave and that her only refuge would be with her mother in Saigon.

Meanwhile she was facing another dilemma, one that conflicted with her maternal instincts. An American sergeant who had worked at the Eighth Field Hospital was interested in adopting a Vietnamese child. He had seen little Jimmie and could not forget him. When he learned that the boy was fatherless, he asked Nga for permission to adopt him. Nga knew that if the way opened for her to marry Charles, in all probability she would not be able to take Jimmy with her. Thus she had to plan for his future. Adoption into a good family might be the best for him. So with many misgivings and tears Nga finally allowed her child to be taken. Jimmie was taken to the United States and there joined a family with several children.

Nga returned to Saigon a few months before her new baby was expected. Her applications were still being processed.

Charles wrote her that he was doing whatever was possible for them to be together soon. But in the meantime life was hard for Nga. She could not find any work because of her pregnancy. Her mother, with whom she was staying, bitterly resented her having given up Jimmie, and could not understand that it was best for everyone. After some weeks, Nga became friendly with some Mennonite missionaries in Saigon, and went to live in their home until her baby girl was born.

One week before the birth of the baby, Charles returned. He had been able to get the papers and they were married. He had to leave immediately but before doing so he made arrangements for her to follow. Nga traveled to the States with a month-old baby. How I prayed that her life in a new land, with a new family, amidst people of different ways, would be a happy one.

One Monday morning in the midst of a hectic clinic, a young man walked in with one hand bound up in dirty blood-soaked rags. He told us that the day before he had caught it in the motor of his boat. It was his right hand and it required extensive repair by Dr. Yoder. He was a fisherman. He faced his ordeal with calm curiosity and proved to be an excellent patient.

One day, before we thought him quite ready for discharge, he came and asked for permission to go home. He promised us that once his hand was healed, he would return and take us on a lobster fishing trip the likes of which we had never experienced. Some men from his village came for him with his boat, and we went to the shore to watch him depart. It was a great and beautiful sight to watch this strong, rugged fisherman putting out to sea, for he seemed to be so much a part of it. Standing in the bow, he waved gaily back to us. He was grateful for the help given to him.

118

Duc was true to his word. On a Sunday, weeks later, he came for us in his motorboat. We took off, heading over the sparkling sea toward some islands far out, with sun, wind, and clear blue skies about us. The water was so transparent that one could trace the patterns of the coral beneath. We found an island out of the path of the wind where the sea seemed smooth as glass. One of Duc's friends, also a fine swimmer, dove overboard, a harpoon in his hand. There was not a ripple as he passed through the water. The boat followed the man's body and we watched as he speared a lobster with incredible swiftness and dexterity. My inexperienced eyes had never seen such a feat of skill. The diver rose to the surface and rejoined us, face dripping and grinning, laughter in his eyes, and a very large lobster firmly impaled on his harpoon. This was the first of many and varied kinds of sea creatures that were caught that day. At noon we beached on the island, built a fire, and cooked our meal. It was a stew that included puffer fish, squid, sea snake, hermit crabs, and clams, as well as lobster—no sharks, however. It was a meal delicious beyond belief. It was followed by an afternoon of swimming and lazy sunning. We returned to the Chan-Y-Vien, tired and sunburned, having had a wonderful day.

Nam, whose foot was saved by Dr. Walton, was another fisherman friend. One day when I returned to the Chan-Y-Vien after a trip to town, Hai came running to meet me.

"Come quickly," he said, "and see Nam's gift." He led the way into the hospital, where Nam and his son stood waiting, both of them smiling happily. There, placed on my desk in the clinic, was a magnificent lamp that Nam had made for me.

As proudly as if he were exhibiting his firstborn son, the fisherman directed Hai to plug in the cord and turn on the lamp. I gasped with delight. In the glow of the soft light it was beautiful. It had been carefully and painstakingly made from a huge spread of snow-white finger coral that he had artfully cemented onto a heavy pottery jar. With my two arms I could barely have reached around its circumference.

My pleasure was real and my face must have revealed it. Finally I blurted out in Vietnamese a sorely inadequate thank you. "It is a small gift to bring so much happiness," he replied.

The Yoders came in then and were deeply impressed by Nam's gift to me. Nam had given both Dr. Walton and Dr. Yoder shell lamps when he left the hospital but they were not as magnificent as this. Later Nam confided to me that he had bought those lamps but that for me he wanted to make one with coral he had brought up from the sea himself.

Dr. Yoder asked me to translate to Nam that the lamp was so beautiful that he should go into business as a lamp-maker. Nam shook his head and answered that, like his father, he was a man of the sea. "Soon I will go back and teach my son the ways of a fisherman," he told the doctor. "It is an honor to our fathers to do the work we have learned from them."

13

THE MAJORITY OF the American population of Nhatrang were members of the military. We civilians, in the minority, were often included in their social activities.

When time and weather permitted, we got together for boating and swimming parties, picnics on the beach and tennis matches on the courts in the MAAG compound and at the Eighth Field Hospital. The shortage of American women —only a few senior MAAG officers had their wives with them in Nhatrang—predictably resulted in increased popularity at these outings for the Army nurses, Phyllis, and myself.

Shortly after Easter, there was a flurry of excitement among the Americans. One of the MAAG officers, a young captain who had been in Nhatrang for a year, was marrying an American civilian nurse who was a member of the newly established U.S.O.M. surgical team sent from Washington to serve at the Province Hospital. The couple had been dating for only a few months, but because the groom's duty tour was ending, they decided to be married and leave together.

The wedding was planned for nine o'clock in the morning in the chapel on the compound of the Eighth Field Hospital. The early hour was chosen partly because it was cooler than later in the day, and partly so that a leisurely wedding breakfast could be held before the bride and groom left on the two o'clock plane for Saigon.

Women guests at the wedding wore sheer sleeveless dresses and, knowing the small chapel would be hot and stuffy even at that hour, carried fans. The formality of the occasion demanded that the men, except for the few civilians, wear regulation tropical uniforms, which included snug-fitting jackets. Normally, when off duty, all Army men dressed in civilian sports clothes that rarely included a coat.

Some of the most beautiful Dalat roses I have ever seen decorated the altar but, like the uniformed guests, they soon wilted from the heat.

On the stroke of nine, the groom and best man took their places. A lieutenant standing beside the organ signaled the organist to start playing—she was a young married friend of the couple, soon to become a mother. With the appropriate chords from *Lohengrin*, the bride, on the arm of her groom's commanding officer, started down the aisle. She wore a white lace dress and a small hat and carried a bouquet of white roses. The ceremony went off without a hitch—no misplaced wedding ring or undue nervousness on the part of either the bride or groom.

Afterward, outside the chapel, rose petals and rice were tossed at the happy couple. With much mock formality a "guard of honor" assisted the newlyweds and their attendents into gaily decorated *xich-los* that would take them to their wedding reception. At once a procession formed behind the bridal party. It included jeeps, half-ton trucks, several Land-Rovers and Volkswagens—all loaded down with cheering guests. Along the route, horns went full blast, causing Vietnamese, unfamiliar with this custom, to stop and stare—and then to laugh.

Reaching the Pacific Hotel, one of Nhatrang's highest buildings, everyone piled out of the assorted vehicles and queued up to follow the bridal couple to the roof garden. The hotel, which had been leased as a billet for American officers, fronted on a stretch of the beach. The top floor, where the wedding breakfast was held, had been converted into an officer's club, and it commanded a sweeping view of the beach and the sea.

When the last guest had passed through the reception line, the bride cut the cake—a truly monumental example of the skill of the chief baker at the Eighth Field Hospital, and everyone sat down to an elaborate brunch.

The only other wedding I attended in Vietnam was Mimmie's a few months later. Although both were Christian weddings, the contrast between them was considerable. Mimmie was dressed in the standard Vietnamese *ao-dai*. She wore a white lace tunic over a pale pink one; and, of course, the usual white satin trousers. On her head she wore a tall seed-pearl crown from which her veil fell to her shoulders. The young man Mimmie married was the son of a pastor and his father acted as best man during the ceremony, which was held at the Bible School chapel.

The ceremony itself was not unlike the usual Christian ceremony except for the fact that it was conducted in Vietnamese. At its conclusion, we remained in the chapel for half an hour longer while the pastor read congratulatory telegrams.

Mimmie's wedding reception took place in Nhatrang's "number one" Chinese restaurant. There were over fifty guests and gaiety reigned, as on such happy occasions everywhere. The bride, her close friends, and younger brothers and sisters had their banquet in a small room adjoining a larger one where the guests were. After the banquet the bridal couple, accompanied by Mimmie's father, went from table to table, laughing and talking with all of the guests. Mimmie was radiant. Later, her two small sisters entertained with a traditional Vietnamese children's dance, and she sang with them in a sweet clear voice.

When it came time to say goodbye to Mimmie and wish her unbounded happiness, I did so with a real sense of personal loss. She was a wonderful girl and had given so much of herself in the months she had worked with us. We had become attached to each other and I knew I would miss her.

After the wedding I went back, changed into my uniform, and found an unexpected problem waiting for me at the hospital's back door. One of our young patients at that time was a young woman fatally ill with cancer of the bladder. I was used to the fact that the Vietnamese preferred to have death occur at home rather than in the hospital, even if we could make the last days and hours more comfortable for the patient. So I was annoyed but not at all surprised to have the young woman's mother announce that she was going to take her daughter, still hemorrhaging, home. Indeed, the small car she had already hired at great expense was waiting for its passengers at that moment. Unfortunately, I had no choice but to capitulate.

Most Vietnamese are Buddhists, but not of the same sect as in India, Burma, Thailand, Cambodia, and Laos. The Vietnamese practice is a variation of Mahayana or Greater

Vehicle Buddhism as practiced in China and Japan. It is a liberal and tolerant branch of the religion, substantially influenced by Confucianism and Taoism due to centuries of contact with China. Animism and ancestor worship are two distinctive characteristics of what is actually more of a popular folk religion than a formal theology.

An outgrowth of this reverence for deceased members of one's family is the reverence for one's elders and fidelity to one's relatives. The latter principle is so strongly ingrained that divorce and abandonment of children are virtually nonexistent. Attendance at religious ceremonies is not required and there is no compulsory period of priesthood for men, as is demanded in the Hinayana or Lesser Vehicle Buddhism of India and elsewhere in Southeast Asia.

Although long periods of mourning and elaborate cremation rites prevail among Buddhists in these countries, in Vietnam the dead are buried quickly. It is believed that if death takes place away from home the spirit of the deceased will wander indefinitely. Respecting this, we always tried to comply with family wishes to have death occur at home, and there had been many times when I, against my better medical judgment, had to let a dying patient leave the hospital. Sometimes, when a patient's family could not provide a conveyance, and when they insisted that the patient be brought home to die, it devolved upon us to provide transportation. I had made these trips, with a dying patient and perhaps one or more relatives behind me in the Land-Rover, on frequent occasions. But there was one drive into the hinterlands on such a mission that I shall never forget.

It began when a boy of seventeen stricken with cirrhosis of the liver, lapsed into a coma after he had been in the hospital several weeks. We knew the end was near and I agreed to take the boy and his mother to their home in a farming area. Hai went with me.

I was not familiar with this particular rural district, so while I drove, the mother, sitting in the rear of the Land-Rover with her son, called out which roads we should take.

For the last leg of the hour-long journey we drove along the top of a narrow dirt dike that separated two rice fields. With little clearance on each side, I drove in low gear and with great care. Where the flooded rice paddies did not abut the dike, there were deep muddy irrigation ditches. We reached the patient's home without incident. But I could not yet draw a deep breath of relief. We still had the return journey ahead of us.

After leaving the boy and his mother I turned around and Hai and I began to retrace our steps. We drove again along the narrow dike road. It was just my luck, when passing one of the ditches between the rice paddies, to have a water buffalo suddenly heave itself out of the mire and start across the dike directly in front of the car. I braked quickly and, hoping to avoid the animal, instinctively gave the wheel a slight turn. The beast continued on his lumbering way unharmed, but the Rover slid down the embankment. It ended up at a crazy angle, half in and half out of the ditch, with slime leaking into the driver's seat. Hai and I scrambled out on the opposite side of the front seat and surveyed the damage. Farmers and their families from the nearby hamlet came running. The men promptly offered advice and assistance. They brought logs and, standing knee deep in the ditch, tried to pry the Land-Rover loose. The heavy vehicle resisted their efforts, obstinately settling back into an even more precarious position.

Just as the farmers were conferring among themselves

about what steps should be taken next and Hai and I were looking at each other, torn between helpless anger at our frustrating situation and helpless laughter at the ludicrous position of the old car, we saw coming toward us, in single file along the dike, a company of Vietnamese soldiers. They were all dressed in camouflage uniforms, with camouflage helmets, and each man carried a rifle except for the lead soldier and one in the rear, who carried walkie-talkies. All the men kept on marching past us, looking at us only out of the corners of their eyes. At the very end of the line marched a jaunty sergeant, carrying a swagger stick. He pulled up sharply when he saw us, grabbed a walkie-talkie and ordered his men to halt. In passable English, the sergeant politely turned to me and expressed dismay at our plight. He said he would try to solve our problem.

Transmitting his orders by walkie-talkie, he told his men to about-face and line up at attention. After explaining my predicament he told them to stack arms and strip. They did so, folding their garments neatly and placing them in separate piles in one small dry area at the edge of the road. In an instant they were wearing nothing but their shorts. Deploying a third of the men to the upper end of the Rover, the sergeant sent the rest with the farmers' logs below to place the timbers under the chassis. Sheer manpower did the rest: at the command to "lift" the men picked up the vehicle and swung it back onto the dike.

Cheers went up from the villagers and from Hai and me. The sergeant beamed. While his men got back into uniform and retrieved their arms he chatted with me. He was quite nonchalant about the incident. He said he knew from my white uniform that I was a nurse, so he had felt dutybound to help me. He suggested that I not take this route along the dike but that I turn off onto a road that passed through the village from which the farmers had come. Although it was a longer route, it was a better road.

Hai's eyes had been popping out while our rescue took place—he was so impressed with the sergeant's efficiency and courtesy to me. I thanked the sergeant and he gave me a snappy salute. Little Hai returned the salute as briskly as he could. Then, placing his swagger stick jauntily against his trousers, the sergeant gave his men the order to march, and away went our benefactors.

For all its seriousness—goodness knows how long the Land-Rover might have remained mired in that ditch—the affair was not without humor. It was hard not to laugh at the sight of the soldiers dutifully stripping for action. But mostly I was glad that neither the dying boy nor his mother were involved in the mishap, that they were already in their simple two-room house beside a rice field. At least my mission had been accomplished before our accident took place.

In the spring of 1963 we were jolted by official notification that the outskirts of Nhatrang, including the Chan-Y-Vien and the surrounding area, were to come under the strategic hamlet program, the plan promoted by the government of Premier Diem to fortify all rural settlements as a defense against guerrilla attack. A hamlet was considered to be a cluster of neighboring houses. Not only were the hamlets to be fenced in, but each individual house within the hamlet was to have a fence built at the perimeter of its property as well. To this day, I do not know to which hamlet the Chan-Y-Vien was supposed to belong, but that is beside the point; the hospital was expected to conform to the order and erect fences around its compound. This edict also resulted in the placing of our fortified hamlet "off limits" to American Army personnel. We could continue to take patients to the Eighth

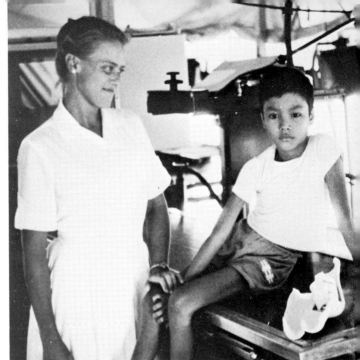

With Phi in the X-ray room at the Eighth Field Hospital after the cast was removed from his knee.

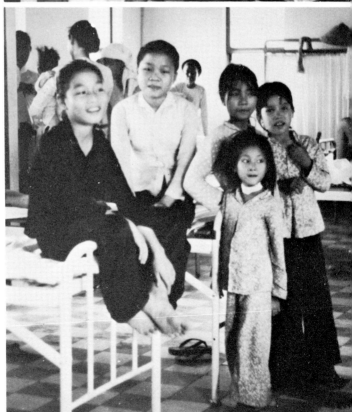

Patients and visitors in the ward of the Chan-Y-Vien.

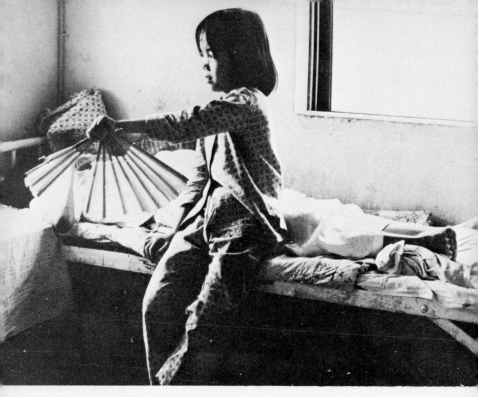

Tragic portrait of mother and child.

Ba Ba's husband, our night watchman, and his children.

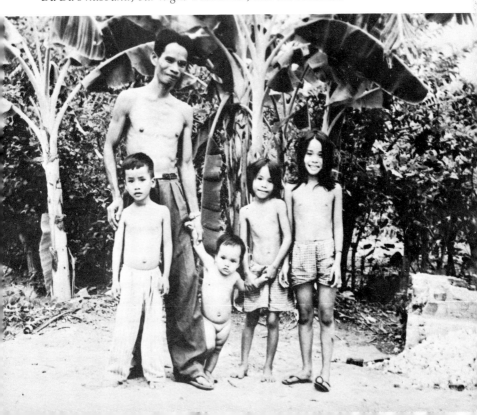

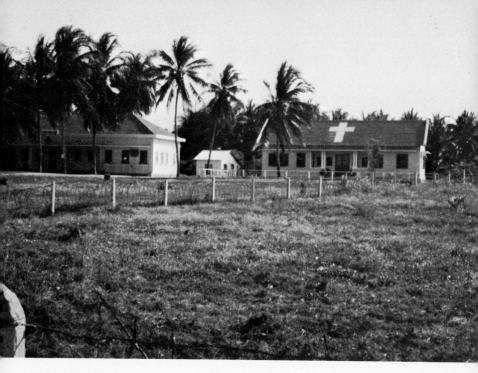

The Chan-Y-Vien and the bungalow.

The verandah of the Chan-Y-Vien
seen at a quiet hour . . . and crowded
with patients lined up for clinic.

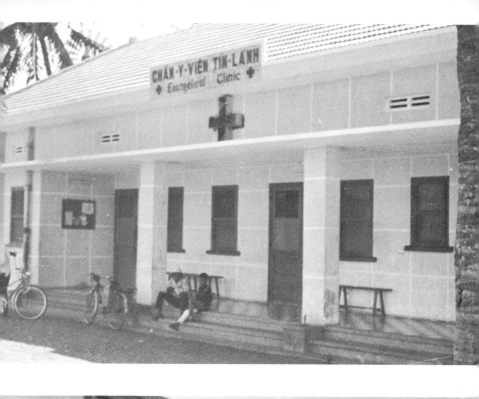

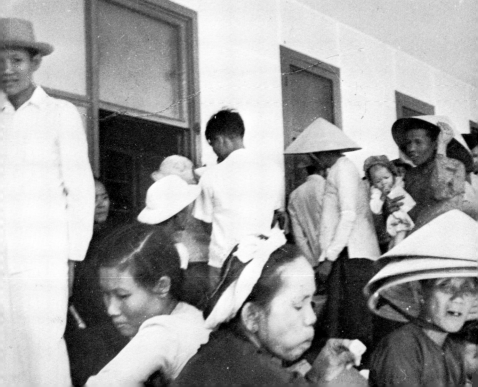

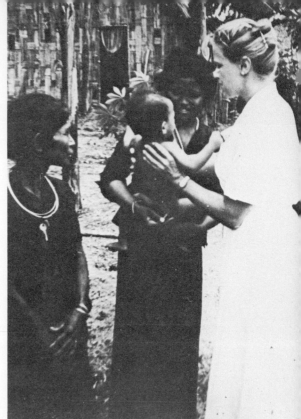

*With the
hill people
of Phuoc Luong.*

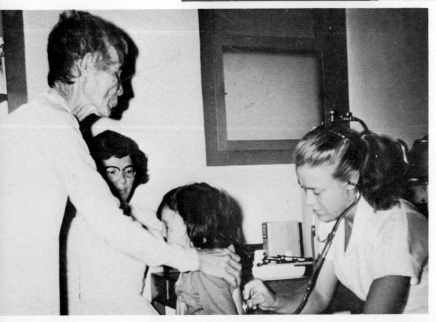

A routine examination in the clinic of the Chan-Y-Vien.

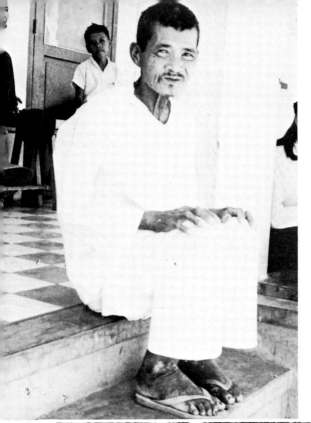

*San, about 70;
a tubercular
patient.*

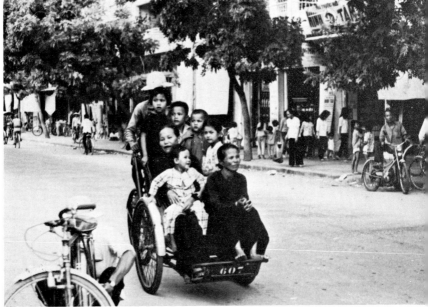

A crowded xich-lo in Nhatrang.

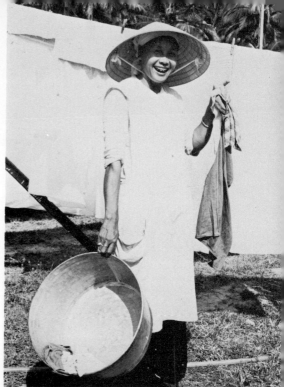

Ba Ba holding the basin that was used for sounding the alarm.

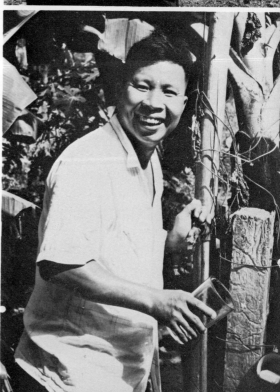

Anh Ba.

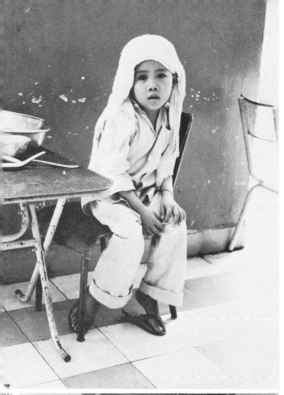

Patients frequently covered their heads with towels as protection against the "poison winds."

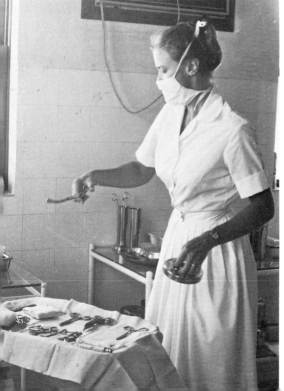

Phyllis took this picture of me laying out sterile instruments.

Mothers of patients giving their children the mid-day meal.

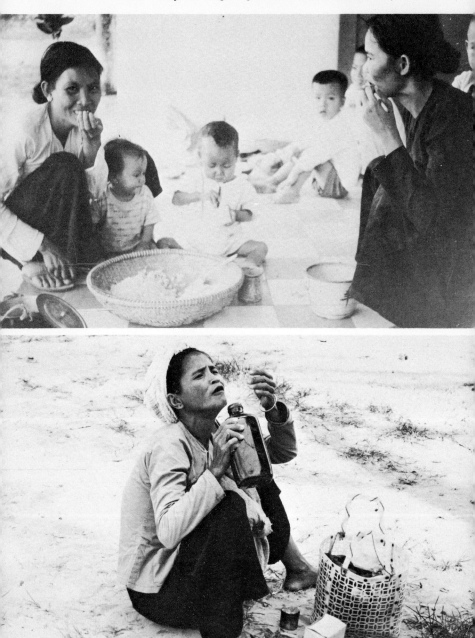

This woman was given pills at the dispensary. Although there was no urgency about her taking them, she sat right down outside the hospital, and is seen here about to begin her medication.

Vendors and patients out front.

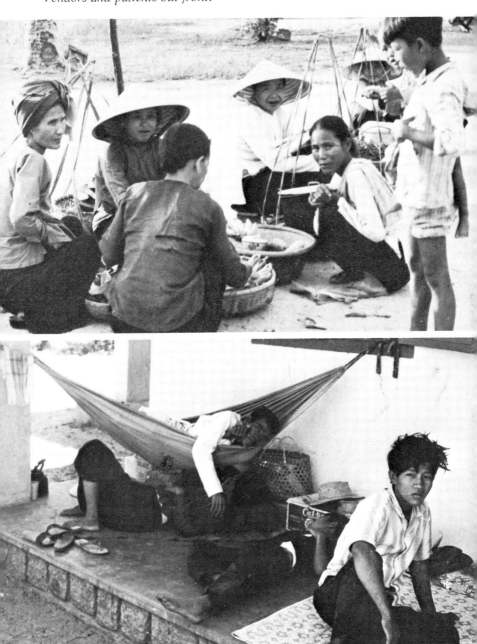

*When all the beds were filled, patients
slept outside in hammocks or on straw mats.*

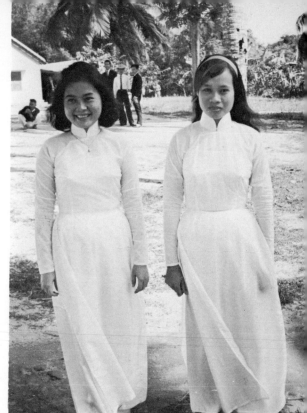

*These girls in their
traditional ao-dais
are hospital aides.*

*Mimmie's wedding in
the Bible School chapel.*

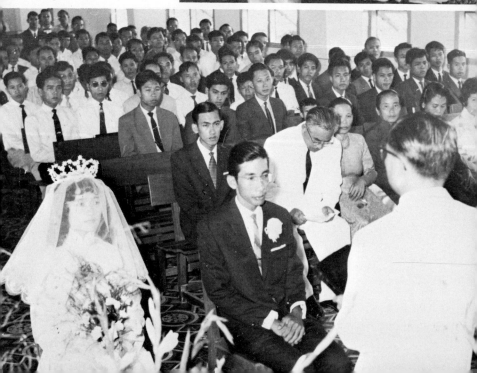

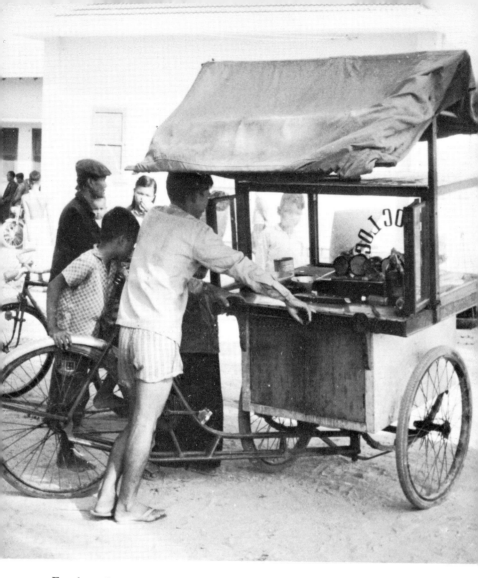

Food vendors near the hospital.

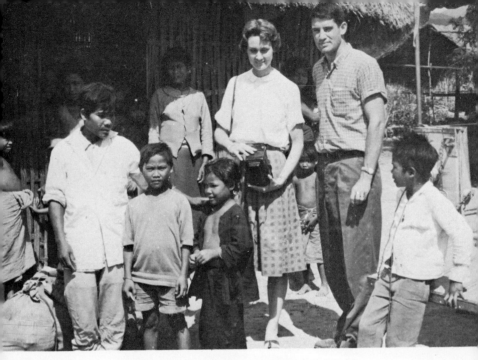

Dr. Yoder, Phyllis, and the Land-Rover at the Phuoc Luong resettlement village.

Dr. Yoder examining a patient at the resettlement village.

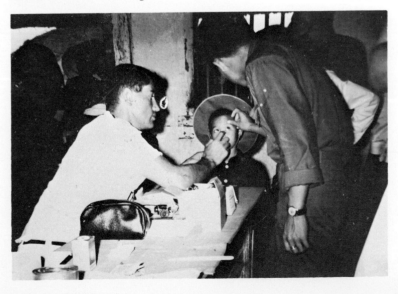

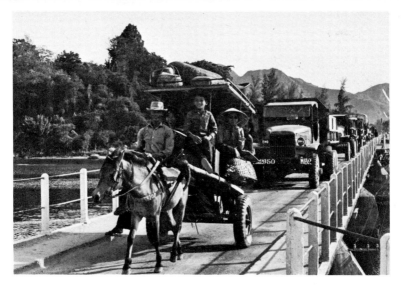

The bridge on which the Land-Rover broke down.

*The crowd that came out
to watch Phi arrive by helicopter.*

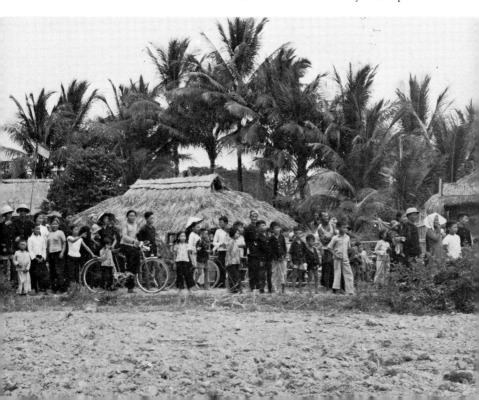

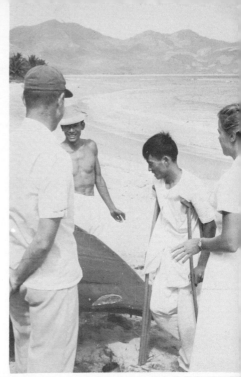

Dr. Walton, Chao, Nam, and myself examining the hull of the Duc-Tin.

Chao and Anh Ba on the Duc-Tin.

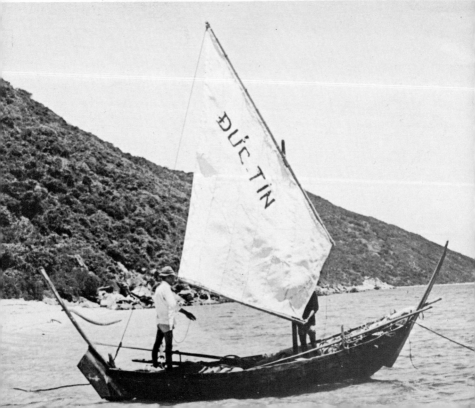

Field Hospital and the Province Hospital for X-rays, laboratory tests, and major surgery, but if the government order were strictly enforced Army doctors would not be able to hold consultations with Dr. Yoder at the Chan-Y-Vien.

Our all-Vietnamese Board of Directors explained further that each person or householder would be held personally responsible if anyone were caught crossing his private property during the night. They feared that, if we did not comply with these regulations, Dr. Yoder, Phyllis, and I might be kidnapped by the Vietcong as the staff at the Banmethuot leprosarium had been. We understood these fears, which were based on their belief that the Vietcong were in great need of trained medical personnel. But we felt confident that the best guarantee of safety would be for us to continue to live and work as naturally and normally as always.

It happened that the Army doctors, although continuing to come to our hospital for consultations, found it necessary to reduce the number of their visits because of their own increased work load. This met with the approval of our board of directors, who felt that too many vehicles marked with Army insignia parked outside the Chan-Y-Vien might attract unfavorable attention. But the Yoders and I came and went day and night and never felt the slightest cause for concern.

Another element in the fortified hamlet program was an alarm system. Each householder within the controlled areas was expected to have on hand pails and tin cans which could be pounded on with sticks if suspicious characters or strangers were seen lurking in the night.

One evening after the Yoders and I had finished dinner and were sitting out on the back stairs where there was a breeze, talking about nothing much in particular, we heard sounds of metallic banging in the distance. It was scarcely nine o'clock—the time set for the closing and locking of the gates at each end of the dirt road that ran by our compound. We listened for a few seconds. Then I jumped up and ran into the kitchen to get Anh Ba's laundry tub and a broom. With the implements in hand, I rejoined the Yoders and at once smacked the broom handle against the tub.

In the distance we could hear a similar commotion coming from other houses, punctuated by occasional shouts and hoots of laughter. When we heard the commotion, Hai came running over from the hospital to join in the fun. Soon we were all giggling together over the racket. When we stopped banging, we heard answering noises from the direction of Anh Tin's house close by. We listened to his tattoo, then answered with another of our own. He replied with a rhythmic beat; I imitated it. Soon we were echoing each other's syncopation. After about five minutes of this Phyllis dubbed me "Chief Minister of Defense." Then she and the doctor and I, still laughing, went inside. We gave Hai some cookies with strict orders to share them with the other children at the hospital and then went to bed.

The morning after the "big band" Anh Ba presented us with a small, shiny, black puppy. He said he was sure the cuddly little animal would grow up to be a fine watchdog. We named her Missy and in addition to becoming a lovable pet, she did in time become quite a formidable protector.

Later during the day of Missy's arrival, we were given four plump geese by Vietnamese friends who explained that the unfriendly birds with their raucous honking would be a good alarm system if we were ever bothered by intruders. We accepted this kindly gesture in the spirit in which it was made. But those geese were absolutely useless; they slept all night. And when Thanksgiving came we decided that it would be more practical to eat them than to keep them. This

130

was in no sense construed as cruelty to feathered friends; geese are favored fare with the Vietnamese.

The gate-closing alarm was repeated the following evening, and the evening after that, and was considered by everyone to be a great joke on the authorities. Had there been real cause for an alarm, it is likely that nobody would have known it. But after about a week the joke palled and the nightly alarm was seldom heard after that.

14

We never found out whether any of the drum-beating episodes was a genuine alarm. Dr. Yoder spoke with Vietnamese officials from time to time, but he was usually unable to learn if there really had been Vietcong activity or not. Either they didn't know or they were unwilling to reveal what was going on. Vietnamese civilians never mentioned any incidents to us; they did not usually discuss anything that had to do with the war. And the American Army officers we spoke to were uncertain about whether there actually was Vietcong activity in our immediate vicinity.

Meanwhile, from listening to the nightly news roundup broadcast from Manila by the Voice of America, we learned of stepped up military activity by Vietnamese forces. It was reported that in the South, especially in the Mekong Delta region where much Vietcong action took place, an increasing number of American military advisers attached to Viet-

mission by Washington to return fire and that combat troops would be sent into Vietnam.

Late in May Phyllis' parents arrived from Hue on their way back to the States. They brought news of a disturbing event that had taken place there two weeks earlier and about which we had heard only fragmentary reports. There had been bloodshed in the city during the annual celebration of Buddha's birthday. Since the population there was about 90 per cent Buddhist, the holiday was normally a significant occasion. Shortly before the festivities were to begin an order was issued by the predominantly Catholic Diem government in Saigon that no Buddhist flags were to fly on that day. As a result of bitter protests this order was rescinded, but the government then refused to permit scheduled radio time for speeches and songs in honor of the holiday.

That evening a large crowd gathered outside the radio station. They protested that the refusal of air time constituted a denial of religious freedom. Government police were summoned and, without making any attempt to disperse the crowd, charged into it and opened fire. It was said that at least eight people were killed.

The following day there was more trouble. Buddhists came from many miles away to take part in the mass funeral services arranged for the victims of the preceding evening. The procession that afternoon was long and noisy, with many of the mourners shouting anti-Catholic and anti-government slogans. Overhead, American helicopters carrying government policemen buzzed the enormous crowd. In return, the marchers called out for them to drop their bombs. The chant, "We are not afraid to die," spread through the crowd and before long it became hysterical with outrage.

Phyllis' father told us that one of the results of this incident was even greater popular hostility against the already hated Diem regime. The people looking overhead had seen American-made helicopters that carried Vietnamese crews but were flown by American pilots. The inevitable conclusion was that American policy condoned and supported the Diem government's suppression of religious freedom and was thus indirectly responsible for the deaths that had occured.

As matters stood in Hue, it was widely believed that an open revolt by the local Buddhists could be expected at any time. The military conflict in South Vietnam was declared a "war of religious persecution."

Although we had been hearing the Voice of America broadcasts with regularity, we had not heard any mention of the trouble in Hue until several days later. We concluded that the Saigon government had banned the release of any information and that the United States had agreed to keep the whole thing quiet. We had first learned of the situation in the northern city from the people working for us. Their information most probably originated with travelers coming from Hue, who told friends, who told friends. We learned that, somewhat later, the Vietnamese radio did broadcast some of this news.

So far in Nhatrang there had been no Buddhist demonstrations, or even rumors of discontent. The city was about evenly divided between Catholics and Buddhists although the surrounding rural areas were predominantly Buddhist. Everyone went about his business as usual. For all we knew, we could have been living in the most peaceful country on earth. All we wished was that this could have been truly so.

Since the Buddhist cemetery was beyond the narrow bridges across the two channels of the Nhatrang river and not too many miles from our hospital, we were often delayed on the one-lane spans by funeral processions when trying to get to and from the city. One afternoon when I was returning from the Eighth Field Hospital and was starting to drive over the first bridge, I saw in the rear-view mirror that a funeral procession was about to catch up with the Land-Rover. I at once stepped on the gas. The motor coughed and threatened to quit. A few more feet and the truck stopped coughing and came to a standstill. I had five patients with me—three children who had been X-rayed and two post-operative cases who had undergone surgery only that morning. Hai was, as usual, along for the ride. I was furious about the breakdown—even though it occurred at a turnout in the road which would at least permit the funeral procession and other following traffic to pass us.

From previous experience I knew that a vapor lock had silenced the engine and there was nothing to do but wait until the metal cooled off; this might take from 10 to 20 minutes and I'd be sure to be caught behind the procession on the second bridge. Goodness only knew when I'd get the patients back to the Chan-Y-Vien; the children were already restive and one of the surgical cases complained about being thirsty. If only a vendor of fruit ices had been near; but all I saw was the funeral procession headed directly toward us. I hoped the mourners would not be unduly distracted by the sight of an obviously Western woman seated in a dilapidated truck, with several wide-eyed children craning their necks out the back.

At the head of the procession several saffron-robed Buddhist monks rode with bowed heads, each in a *xich-lo* by himself. Because of the presence of more than one monk, I knew that this was the funeral either of another monk or of some person of more than ordinary wealth and distinction. Then there came a detachment of empty *xich-los*, each with a banner on a pole. The banners were white with black Chinese characters, said to be auspicious adages which related to a happy future for the deceased.

Three walking musicians were next. One slowly hit a large deep-sounding drum. The other two, in the same cadence, struck their gongs with padded hammers.

Behind them was the black hearse pulled by six men, all wearing black knickers and shirts. A picture of the deceased, garlanded with flowers, was attached to the front of the hearse. Inside rested the coffin with two candles burning on the scarlet lid. Flowers were heaped around the plain wooden box. Beside the hearse walked the oldest son or brother dressed in a long white tunic with a black armband.

Buddhist friends, including several devout elderly ladies attired in gray who held their hands in an attitude of prayer, walked behind the funeral car. Other family members and friends rode in buses which were decorated with more banners and streamers of black crepe. A number of these people stared openly at me.

I gave the crawling procession half an hour to cross the bridge and be on the highway that traversed the island in the middle of the river. Then I stepped on the starter. The engine caught and off we roared. With relief I passed the procession when it was almost at the end of the road, just in time to reach the second bridge. I was within five feet of being across the second bridge when a tire blew. The bridge guard came over and offered sympathy, explaining that he was on duty and couldn't help. There was no one else in sight. I couldn't let the truck block the oncoming procession, so I got out, gave it a push, then hopped in and steered it down the incline and off to one side. Now the usual crowd of onlookers appeared, coming from all directions. The Land-Rover and I were a familiar sight, and our present predicament was more cause for amusement than concern. As was customary, everybody laughed and, there being nothing else to do, I in my stained and crumpled uniform laughed most of all. I was somewhat puzzled to discover that there was no spare tire. But I decided that, if I sat there long enough, somebody who knew me would come along.

Sure enough, after the funeral procession passed—the mourners, staring, surely thought they were seeing double—along came an Army jeep. The G.I.s stopped and I told them my troubles. We decided that, first of all, the patients must be taken to the Chan-Y-Vien. Gently they transferred the two surgery cases to the back of the jeep and packed the children up in front.

Hai stayed with me until the jeep returned. The G.I.s said they'd send someone from the motor pool at the base out with a tire. They had not realized that the hospital's transportation facilities depended entirely on the Land-Rover, which by then was obviously just about done for.

Taking Hai and me up the hill in the jeep, the G.I.s said over and over that the hospital needed a new truck—and maybe if they thought long enough they might find a way to get us one.

When I got back at last I ranted on and on to Phyllis about my misadventures with the dilapidated vehicle. "And the last straw was not having a spare tire," I finally concluded.

"Just calm down now," she laughed. "I had a blowout this morning and had to use the spare. I didn't get a chance to tell you. Don't complain to me about that car!"

About a week later a group of soldiers came to take snapshots of the hospital. They said the pictures would be used on posters announcing a softball game to raise some of the money they were collecting for our new truck.

We knew that both officers and men in the various Army installations around town were always conducting a fund drive for a worthy purpose—but we were stunned, and of course very grateful, for this unexpected generosity.

Hai declared that seeing the same funeral procession twice had brought the good luck.

Eventually other contributers were enlisted as well. Phyllis' parents took up a collection among their friends back in Goshen, Indiana, and several wealthy Vietnamese, including a baker in Saigon, also helped the G.I.s reach their goal.

15

I HAD BEEN IN Vietnam almost a year and a half. Little by little I was beginning to feel wiser and tougher.

The surprise and disappointment I had felt when I first arrived at the Chan-Y-Vien to find only a handful of ward- and outpatients was becoming something of a standing joke. Now there were usually at least 200 clinic patients a day and often more. And there were never fewer than 30 patients in the ward—more than twice its capacity—at any one time. It became customary to put two or three sick children in one bed and to put the overflow of adult patients on hammocks, stretchers, or on grass mats on the floor. If two children were supposed to be sharing a bed, there would also be two mothers on or near that bed taking care of their respective children. A baby might occupy a little hammock strung between the bedposts while the mother crouched on a mat. Those who slept on the floor were happiest since most of them were afraid of falling out of a hospital bed. But nursing them was a real problem for us since it involved a lot of bending and squatting and being careful not to step on outstretched hands during the night. After a while Phyllis and I automatically looked under the beds as well as on them for our patients.

As the ward began to look less and less like its Western counterparts, I more and more appreciated the Chan-Y-Vien operating room, which even with maximum usage was a haven of professional calm. We were still not equipped for major surgery, but Dr. Yoder took real advantage of our facilities for minor operations. Patients came from as far away as Hue in the north and even Saigon, brought by his reputation for eye surgery. He set aside Wednesdays and Saturdays for entropion and cataract operations and helped literally hundreds of people. He even trained our best aide, Anh Tin, to do entropions.

Under Dr. Yoder's guidance our Vietnamese hospital staff was becoming increasingly competent. They were able to perform such nursing chores as changing intravenous bottles and dressings and giving medication and injections—of course, under supervision.

In turn, I was often called on to perform medical duties quite beyond those normally expected of a nurse. I learned to detect the symptoms of the most prevalent diseases: tuberculosis, liver ailments, and stomach and kidney malfunctioning. At one point I also learned how to extract teeth, but I never enjoyed the procedure enough to achieve proficiency in it. My extractions were restricted to that last loose tooth left in the mouth of an old lady, which I could pull without the use of instruments. But lancing and treating external abcesses became commonplace.

Dr. Yoder's first responsibility was to the critically ill,

whether they were in the ward or the outpatient clinic. As the number of patients increased, caring for them and maintaining his heavy surgery schedule took almost all of his time. Consequently many diagnostic and other non-nursing jobs became mine. With no assisting doctor available, Dr. Yoder just had to make the most of his chief nurse's abilities.

There was now talk of adding a new wing to the Chan-Y-Vien to accommodate the additional patients. We had already requested that the Mennonite Central Committee expand our professional staff, but they were having trouble recruiting doctors and nurses, partly because of the worsening political and military situation.

Because of the crowded ward, we tried to discourage maternity cases and took only first births or women who had a history of difficulty in childbearing. I would say to a woman, "You've had five babies and never had any trouble. Just go back to the birth house in your village." But we were able to give some prenatal care if they came to us during pregnancy; vitamins were the most important aid we could give them at this time. The complications of childbearing were caused primarily by poor nutrition on the part of the mother. The babies were small by American standards, averaging under six pounds at birth.

Despite our discouraging them, we still had a fair number of deliveries, usually late at night. After one such all-night session I was particularly tired and irritable. I settled the last mother and her infant, cleaned up the operating room, and realized that there was barely an hour left in which I could freshen up and have a quick breakfast before clinic.

Exhausted, I sat at the table in the clinic room, examining people who were queued up, waiting, holding numbers from 1 to 100 to indicate their turn. Children were milling around and curious faces filled the windows that opened onto the verandah. My interpreter sat at the table, too, helping interview the patients. The other assistants stood near the open shelves along one wall where the medicines were "filed"—all those starting with "A" on one shelf, followed by the "B's" and so on. I would write my prescription on a small card which was then passed to one of the aides who would write the information in our permanent record book. Then the others would fill the prescription.

As I forced myself to forget my exhaustion and concentrate on the cases before me, I heard a commotion on the verandah. Even before I looked up I knew that it heralded the arrival of a possible emergency. The crowd parted and two men came in bearing a hammock slung over a pole. Without pausing they came right up to me and dropped their burden at the foot of my examining table. Everyone crowded back into the room behind them, chattering excitedly and ogling the stretcher and its contents. The children clustered on my left to see what was going on. Over the months the patients had developed an unwritten rule: anyone brought in by hammock did not have to wait his turn but could go right to *Co-Y-Ta* to be examined. Anyone brought in this way was sure to be doubled over in a jackknife position in the bottom of the hammock and covered with layers of blankets to protect him from further ravages of the poison wind. I would unfold all the blankets, never sure whether I would find somebody really ill or only someone who wanted instant attention.

But this day the patient brought up to me was clearly a real emergency. His stretcher-bearers, in answer to my questions, told me that he had been ill for more than a week and that for several days his abdomen had been as rigid as a board. Dr. Yoder made a diagnosis of perforated gastric ulcer, which required immediate surgery. Since our facilities were not adequate for such a major procedure, I had to [ ] the man to the Province Hospital.

There were two operating rooms there, but only one U.S.O.M. surgeon. When I told him about the emergency case I had brought with me, he regretted that his own heavy schedule would make it impossible for him to get to this case for quite a while. He offered to call Dr. Tsang, the surgeon at the Eighth Field Hospital, who might be free to come and operate.

I had met Dr. Tsang several times before, when he had been out to the Chan-Y-Vien to look at some of our patients. His reputation was excellent and I liked him. After a thorough examination of the patient, he agreed that only immediate surgery would save the man's life. He invited me to serve as his scrub nurse during the operation.

The job of scrub nurse is a particularly demanding one, requiring calmness, accuracy, and speed, in addition to constantly anticipating the doctor's needs. During a complicated operation there are usually other doctors and nurses present, but the scrub nurse works directly alongside of and with the physician. It was a job I had particularly enjoyed during my student days in New York because of the closeup view I could get of a skillful surgeon at work.

Dr. Tsang's request took me by surprise. My immediate reaction was to say no. I was still tired from my delivery-room activities of the night before and I was afraid I might show that I was out of practice. I hadn't served as a scrub nurse in over two years. But my interest in watching Dr. Tsang in action overruled my qualms. I was, in fact, flattered to be asked.

The operation was a long, painstaking affair and everyone in the room—doctors, nurses, anaesthetist—worked with efficiency. Dr. Tsang managed to inspire the best work pos-

take

m. He was remarkably good and, above all,
⸺rate toward his assistants. But it was his
⸺ed me most. It was the skill of a much
⸺enced man.

⸺tion was over I somehow felt less tired
⸺ before. Dr. Tsang suggested that I join him
ror coffee at one of the beach houses along the road. The
patient would remain in the recovery room for several days
until he could be moved back to the Chan-Y-Vien.

As we relaxed in the nearby beach house, Dr. Tsang
opened the conversation by discussing the surgical procedure that had just been done. He then told me a little about
himself. He was from San Francisco, but had been born and
spent his first seven or eight years in Hong Kong. After coming to the states, his father, a doctor, had opened a successful practice in San Francisco. Dr. Tsang had been a student
at Stanford University and had taken his residency in surgery at the Mayo Clinic. This was not his first trip to the
Orient and he was eager to visit Hong Kong again to see
friends and relations there. I told him I had lived in India for
many years.

He asked why I had come to Vietnam. Giving the answer
that I usually did to this question, I said that I wanted to
travel and get the broad nursing experience one can receive
only in a small, busy hospital. Most people thought I was na-
ïvely idealistic if I simply said I wanted to give help where it
was most needed.

But Dr. Tsang was not the kind of man to whom one could
give simple answers or half truths. I told him of my concern
about the growing war and its effect on the hospital and its
patients, of our problems with insufficient Vietnamese
trained personnel, and of the lack of drugs and supplies.

He listened, speaking little, his face registering what his

146

silence implied—interest, empathy, and understanding of problems we shared. Long after the coffee cups were empty we sat and talked, or simply sat, looking out over the beach to the calm sea and beyond it to the islands and the open horizon. I mentioned my sailboat, the *Duc-Tin*, that had just been given to me by Nam, our fisherman patient. He was delighted and wanted to know more about it. I explained that *Duc-Tin* meant Faith, a name I had chosen for the boat. It was an 18-footer with two masts and a woven bamboo bottom. It was about thirty years old and had been in the family of Nam's mother. It was in Nam's village now, being put in good-as-new condition. I invited him to join me on board as soon as it would be convenient for him, and he accepted the invitation with unconcealed pleasure. He was an ardent fisherman and would be delighted to try his luck on the *Duc-Tin*.

We drove back to the Province Hospital in his jeep for a quick check of the patient, who was doing well and needed only time to recover fully. Then we left the hospital, he to return to the duties he had left undone at the Eighth Field Hospital, and I to drive the now empty truck back to the Chan-Y-Vien. It seemed hours since I had left it.

It was a month before the *Duc-Tin's* hull was recaulked, new sails woven, and the boat put back in the water, and so it was some time before I could make good my sailing invitation. In the meantime on several occasions when a patient from the Chan-Y-Vien was being operated on at the Province Hospital, I scrubbed for Dr. Tsang. This was only partly because I enjoyed this kind of work. Since there was a shortage of nurses familiar with scrub procedures at the Province Hospital, it was frequently a necessity for me to help.

Because the Province Hospital still suffered a shortage of

147

staff personnel and beds, we continued to take our patients back to our own hospital as soon after surgery as possible. Often when the patients had been brought back to the Chan-Y-Vien, Dr. Tsang would make frequent trips to follow each one's progress. In addition to operating on our patients at the Province Hospital, he made arrangements for surgery at the Eighth Field Hospital itself in certain cases where specially trained personnel and equipment were needed.

One day Phyllis confided to me that she and Dr. Yoder were trying to find a child to adopt. Married almost six years, they had so far not had any children of their own. They had already inquired at the orphanage near the Chan-Y-Vien which had been started as a home for the children of ministers killed in the war. Most of the little ones there, however, had one parent still alive and were not available for adoption.

The Yoders knew it would take time to get the legal aspect of an adoption taken care of, and since their term of service was half over, they did not want to delay looking for a child. An acquaintance had suggested that they visit an orphanage in Dalat, and so they planned a long weekend in the cool mountain resort. They would vacation and look for a baby at the same time.

As it happened, the Sunday they were away was perfect for our long deferred day of sailing on the *Duc-Tin*.

Anh-Ba, who had become our cook, did himself proud in preparing us a picnic lunch, being intrigued by this Chinese doctor who he couldn't quite believe was really an American. He cooked up an enormous amount of fried chicken and a marvelous salad of cold rice, pineapples and almonds. He also prepared sandwiches. Before Dr. Tsang arrived, I checked on the patients together with the hospital worker who was on Sunday duty. Things were sufficiently under control for me to feel comfortable about leaving.

While I was preparing the picnic basket, Hai eagerly ran back and forth in the kitchen bringing me things he thought I should have along. He, too, liked the doctor and wanted to be in on as much as he could.

When Dr. Tsang arrived, most of our gear was already on the *Duc-Tin*. Chao, Nam's cousin, and Ba were to be our sailors that day. They had carried down the masts, the sails, the sweeps, the yards of rope, and the floorboards, and by the time Dr. Tsang, Hai and I arrived on the scene, the boat itself was ready. It took several trips between the beach and the shallow sandy area where the boat was anchored to get our lunch and other gear on board. Dr. Tsang brought his fishing equipment, which he usually kept in his jeep just in case he got the chance to use it.

After everything was loaded, I told Hai to wade back to shore, but he looked so crestfallen that I didn't have the heart to insist. I asked Dr. Tsang if he'd mind if the youngster came along. He answered, laughing, that of course he wouldn't mind, if only Hai could keep still while he was fishing. Hai promised solemnly to be good. With a leap and a splash he jumped into the boat—right on top of the picnic basket. Having visions of a crushed dinner, I helped the boy disentangle himself and got him settled near the prow. There he sat, giggling and happy, as we pushed off. Chao and Ba, using the sweeps, rowed until the sails picked up the breeze outside the shelter of the cove, and the *Duc-Tin*, responding to even the slightest tug on the tiller, headed for the islands.

16

It was a perfect day for sailing. The sky was clear, the wind brisk, and the air warmer than usual. Dr. Tsang, Hai, and I sat aft on the floorboards while two fishermen friends of Nam operated the sailboat.

We sped quietly past the rocky headlands and cove beyond the hospital and headed out to sea. The wind whipping by and the hot sun beating down were a welcome balm for sagging spirits. While Dr. Tsang and I basked in the sun, Hai chattered away with the fishermen. When he told what he considered a particularly funny story, he would try desperately to get us to understand the joke, but often my Vietnamese was woefully inadequate for the demands placed on it.

Hai was at his best that day. He was thrilled to be out on the boat with us and apparently had made up his mind to make good his promise to obey. We weren't on board more than half an hour before he was trying to teach us Vietnamese words for various parts of the boat. Dr. Tsang was amused by the boy and before the first hour was up he was giving Hai a lesson in anatomy with the help of a few sticks, stones and some rope. I was content to sit back and watch the changing seascape, the wind filling the sails, and the sun sparkling on the wet deck.

As I looked at my sailing companions, I was suddenly struck by the different appearances presented by the five of us in that boat—myself fair and Nordic-looking, Dr. Tsang with his Chinese features, and Hai, Chao and Ba with their unmistakably Vietnamese faces. With all their similarities, our two sailors were a contrast—Chao tall, slender, open faced, and Ba short, squat, and darker in coloring. Ba's eyes made him look like a rogue, for bilateral entropions that had not been operated on had made him pull out all his lashes, and he squinted against the sun. They were both family men, Chao having two children and Ba eight. I knew Ba's family well; his house was near the Chan-Y-Vien, and sometimes one or two of Ba's children would tag along after their father as he did his chores.

When Hai decided to help Ba with bailing, a constant job on a Vietnamese boat, Dr. Tsang turned to me and began teasing me about my sailing getup. With dark glasses, a patch of adhesive plaster over my nose to avoid sun blisters, and a loose fitting shift over my bathing suit, I was the most covered-up member of the party. In turn I began teasing him about the amount of paraphernalia it took to put him to sea. In addition to his fishing gear, he had come on board with an enormous plastic-lined canvas bag. By way of retort, he dug into the very depths of the bag to produce, of all things, a portable radio and a camera. While I settled even more comfortably against a mast to listen to music over the

Armed Forces Radio Station-Saigon, he took pictures of passing sailboats and motorboats, of Hai, by now asleep in the sun, of Chao and Ba working on the boat, and of the rocky islands we were passing.

Before long I became aware of a pungent, familiar smell. I sat up and saw that we were moving toward an island. By the time the boat docked, the smell was unmistakably that of *nuoc mam*, the omnipresent Vietnamese sauce made from rotting fish. The fishermen had taken us to an island devoted to its manufacture. We thought it might be fun to observe how this sauce was prepared, but the smell, even in the open air, was a bit more than we had bargained for. However, it was a beautiful day, and we were in the mood for adventure, so we set out to explore the island. Hai, Dr. Tsang, and I climbed out of the boat, leaving Chao and Ba on board.

I had never overcome my revulsion to the stench of *nuoc mam*, even though I was quite fond of the taste. I recalled my first experience with the sauce during my first meal at the Chan-Y-Vien, now more than a year and a half before. I told Dr. Tsang how Dr. Dick had urged me to pour it over my food and how surprised I was that something that smelled so awful had tasted so good. I had learned that the name of this sauce, translated literally, meant "whiskers," which symbolized strength.

As we got off the boat, several villagers came over to greet us. They were a happy, carefree group, apparently undisturbed by—very likely inured to—the vile odor that was emitted by their island.

At my inquiry, one of them led us to the home of the villager who seemed to be the owner of the *nuoc mam* factory. It was located in a large room adjoining his house. Here we saw two huge, tall wooden vats filled to the brim with small fish, salt, and brine. This mixture would be allowed to rot for several months, with only the occasional addition of more salt or brine. After the first three months the fluid in the bottom of the vat would be drained off and allowed to settle. This was the best *nuoc mam,* a clear, amber-colored liquid, mild in taste, with, of course, its characteristic odor.

Then more salt and brine would be added to the vats and the mixture would be left to rot for three more months. This six-month mixture was darker in color and stronger in taste and was less prized than the three-month mixture.

Once again salt and brine would be added to the fish remaining in the vats—now more bones and scales than anything else—and after another three months, the nine-month *nuoc mam* would be drained off. This mixture would be the last made from this batch of fish. It was the cheapest and most impure of the three, but because of the low price it was most often used by ordinary village people.

It may be hard to believe, but *nuoc mam* of all three qualities is rich in vitamins and protein. Often the addition of this highly scented liquid to rice is the only thing that saves these people from protein deficiency diseases. Certainly it is the sole source of protein in most Vietnamese diets.

As we were returning to the boat a very old woman, bent, gray, and toothless, came up to me. *"Chao, Co,"* she greeted me. "Hello, Miss." Smiling, she handed me a large and very beautiful pink shell. I thanked her in Vietnamese but couldn't understand what had provoked this lovely and generous gift. Then I looked into her leathery seamed face and recalled that about a year earlier she had tended her infant grandson when he was a patient at the hospital. I asked about the boy and she proudly pointed to a shy toddler playing in front of a nearby house. The child, who had been quite ill, was now the picture of health. I remarked that the child looked sturdy and appeared to be doing well.

As we pulled away from the island I told Dr. Tsang about the case. It was now shortly after noon and the boat was heading for a smaller island, rocky and uninhabited. There we all went swimming and then sat down for our picnic lunch.

While Dr. Tsang kept Hai from plunging into the picnic basket, I unpacked our lunch. Chao and Ba had brought along only rice, and they were delighted when we invited them to share our food. Although most of it was unfamiliar, they were willing to sample everything. We gave them pieces of our sandwiches and small helpings of canned fruit. They seemed particularly fond of peanut butter sandwiches and peaches, as was Hai, who had already developed a taste for these Western goodies. The rice was forgotten and the peanut butter sandwiches disappeared rapidly.

It was mid-afternoon when we returned home. Dr. Tsang had invited me to dinner. We walked up from the beach together and then he left to return to the Eighth Field Hospital. With Hai I went to check things at our hospital. All was quiet in the ward. Most of the patients were asleep and our aides had had very little to do during the day. After finding everything in order, on an impulse I decided to get my hair done. Sitting at the hairdresser's seemed a nice relaxing way to end a leisurely Sunday afternoon.

I left Hai behind to prattle about his adventures, and I drove into town. Kim Hoa's shop was full—Sunday was her busiest day—but she insisted on taking care of me as soon as I entered. While my hair was washed, set, and dried I observed the young women who came and went from the shop. Many of them were very young, perhaps no older than fifteen or sixteen, but all were elaborately dressed and coiffed.

When I first looked around I felt there was something different about these girls, many of whom I had seen before, but I attributed it to the fact that they were all getting themselves beautified, which included getting their fingernails and toenails manicured.

Gradually I became aware of what the change was that I had first merely sensed. It was in their speech. Instead of speaking in the soft, almost whisperlike manner that I was accustomed to, they now spoke loudly and harshly, making sweeping and flamboyant gestures. And these gestures called my attention to the jewelry many of them wore. Although one rarely saw heavily made-up Vietnamese women, some of these girls were now using makeup on their faces. Even their *ao-dais* were different. Many of the tunics were now trimmed with brightly colored sequins on the high collars and long sleeves or were made of fabrics that were different from the traditional.

I realized that this was one more manifestation of the influence of the large number of American soldiers. That presence made itself felt in many ways. Even the price of a *xich-lo* ride was nearly double what it had been before and it was not unusual to see a G.I., perhaps with a local girl friend, sitting in the cab that could hold a whole Vietnamese family.

When I emerged from under Kim Hoa's comb I hardly recognized myself. She had created an elaborate and flamboyant hairdo for me, with a high beehive top and a French twist at the back. She completed her work with Revlon hair spray. I looked taller, older, and infinitely more sophisticated. Although it decidedly wasn't "me," it suited my mood of the moment and I was self-conscious only as a result of the out-of-character transformation.

Hai was standing in the lane waiting for me when I arrived at the hospital. As I drove up he gestured wildly and ran beside me calling out to hurry inside. I raced into the hospital to find Anh Tin at the side of one of the beds. A patient had died in my absence.

I quickly checked the body, that of a seventeen-year-old girl who had had a severe liver ailment, and immediately carried it out to the truck. Her only relative, a sister, had left for the day and was not with her when she died.

Anh Tin volunteered to go with me to help locate her home in one of the market areas of Nhatrang. I can only barely recall what took place between the time I arrived at the hospital and drove into Nhatrang with the girl's body and Anh Tin. Overwhelmed by guilt, I must have been in a state of shock myself. My only thought was to do something, anything, and I must have driven at a furious pace. By the time we arrived in the city, I had calmed down somewhat and made an effort to learn what had happened at the hospital while I was gone. The story I got from Anh Tin was that the patient had suddenly, and apparently inexplicably, gone into a convulsion and died. It had happened without warning, so quickly that nobody was able to do anything before she was gone. I had, I reminded myself, checked her less than three hours earlier and there were no indications of a coming crisis at that time.

Under those circumstances it was unlikely that I could have done anything to save her even if I had been there. But there was always the remote possibility that I might have anticipated it and somehow been able to prevent it. I had left word where I would be, but when the girl went into convulsions there simply wasn't enough time to summon me.

We finally found the little stall where the girl's sister lived, and left the body there. I felt anger at myself as well as guilt and frustration.

156

During the drive back, I reached up to remove something that seemed to be sticking into my head and got my fingers entangled in a mass of strawlike curls. I had completely forgotten about the hairdo. I could imagine what I must have looked like down in the midst of the squalor of that market with my hair done up in this elaborate style as I helped Anh Tin to carry in the stretcher with the body on it. Then I remembered that Dr. Tsang expected me to join him for dinner. In my present mood I just couldn't. I felt I had to get back to the Chan-Y-Vien as quickly as possible. On the way, I stopped at the Eighth Field Hospital and left a message of regret for Dr. Tsang. I was sure he would understand.

When I returned to the hospital I was grateful to find everything in order and that the patients were quietly taking their evening meal. I had neither the physical nor the emotional strength to cope with another crisis.

Anh Ba came to me that evening to say that he was about to cook his own dinner and asked if I would like him to bring me a bowl of it. I was grateful for his arrival, which deprived me of the luxury of wallowing in self-pity. While he disappeared back to his house, I went to the bathroom to compose myself for the evening, which I hoped would be quiet. I caught a glimpse of myself in the mirror and, again, was aghast. I could get neither comb nor brush through the mass of teased and lacquered hair. Finally, giving up, I grabbed my bottle of shampoo and stepped under the shower. The water was cold but I welcomed the chilling shock of it and after several washings and rinsings I finally felt clean again. I braided my damp hair and left it hanging down my back. I put on a cool loose dress and, feeling once more like a human being, ate the dinner Anh Ba brought me. Then I returned to the hospital.

Hai and the patients were pleased that I would remain with them. Hai explained that as long as I was around nobody would be afraid of the wandering spirit of the girl who had died that afternoon. As for me, the best therapy possible was to be busy working with the patients. When I finally got to bed that night, I was so exhausted that every joint and bone in my body ached. Sheer fatigue permitted me the sleep my troubled thoughts might not have otherwise allowed.

Later in the week a whole group of tribespeople appeared on the line for clinic. They came from a village we had visited some time earlier. After Phyllis and I examined them and consulted with Dr. Yoder on whatever problems there were, they all stood around awkwardly. Finally they took the bracelets off their arms and presented them to us. Although the bracelets were just simple rings of brass with some designs scratched into them, we were deeply moved by the gesture. It meant that we were accepted as members of the Koho hill tribe and it signified their gratitude for our medical treatment.

Not too long after that I began preparing for my vacation. My sister Wyva, a social worker, was in India doing research in community development in a leprosy colony. She and I planned to meet in Bangkok to spend our vacation together.

On my way to Bangkok I stopped overnight with the Lichtis in Saigon. It was now several months since I had last been in Saigon and I was shocked to find the city fast becoming an armed camp. Since elections were approaching, security was tighter than it had ever been before. The candidates had all been approved by the Diem government, and since all were Roman Catholics, there were fears of Buddhist demonstrations. There were also stronger defenses set up against Vietcong infiltration. Vehicles entering Saigon were now subject to search. The South Vietnamese had long been required to carry identity cards to prove they weren't members of the Vietcong. Up to now they had rarely been required to present them to police or army officials. But during this trip I found that it had become almost routine for soldiers and plainclothes government agents to demand that shopkeepers, laborers, housewives, students—in fact all civilians—hand over their identity cards for inspection. Failure to comply resulted in immediate arrest.

A strict censorship of newspapers continued to prevail. The government-owned radio station was broadcasting propaganda in favor of the Diem government night and day. No civilian assemblies or parades were permitted, and anyone found making remarks derogatory to Diem chanced imprisonment.

I saw that the presidential palace and all government buildings were under heavy guard. Armed squads patrolled the streets and Army jeeps and trucks with machine guns mounted on them were stationed at strategic points throughout the city. I also noticed that there were more Air Force helicopters and fighter planes flying over the city than ever before.

That evening I commented to Rudi Lichti on the feeling of tension and fear in the air. He said it was constantly increasing. The Diem regime was disliked and mistrusted by its people, and open hostility toward Americans was growing because Washington apparently continued to support Diem.

The brightest point of our evening together was when Rudi announced that work on the addition to the Chan-Y-Vien was scheduled to start before the first of the year and occupancy was expected by spring. Although there had still been no success in recruiting an additional nurse for the hospital, he was hopeful that one would eventually come forth despite the growing political unrest in the country.

Bangkok, in comparison to Saigon, was an oasis of gaiety. The city, with its glittering temples, palaces and exotic bazaars, looked like something out of a fairy tale. The people were happy and gracious and eager to show off their beautiful country. For three days Wyva and I were on a carefree, rejuvenating spree. Then we left for India, and many memories came to life as old haunts were revisited and new places seen. I spent nearly two weeks there and almost forgot the problems that awaited my return.

17

ONE UNFORGETTABLE SATURDAY afternoon shortly after my vacation in India, Hai and I were at the beach having a swim when a cousin of Nam's came running down to say that Nam had just taken a very sick child into the clinic room at the hospital. He asked me to come immediately.

I hurried back to the hospital. The child, a two-and-a-half-year-old boy, was having difficulty breathing. The lymph glands in his neck were extraordinarily large. I left him with Nam and Nam's cousin while I went to get Dr. Yoder at the bungalow. He examined the child in his office adjoining the clinic. Although he could not determine the specific cause of the boy's symptoms, he knew definitely that there was a severe bacterial infection. He began doing a cut-down in order to start intravenous injections of penicillin and strep-tomycin. These highly potent anti-bacterial drugs would work if we were in time. But there was no indication during the several hours we sat beside the stricken infant that he might be reviving. It was near midnight when the child died.

Nam, who had waited on the verandah the whole time, explained that the little one's death would be particularly tragic for his family since his mother had died of typhoid only a few days earlier.

I took Nam and the small body back to the fishing village. Despite the late hour, a light burned in the boy's home. Nam carried the body inside, then came back to express his thanks for the care Dr. Yoder and I had given the child. With amazing composure, Nam said the dead child was his favorite nephew, but since he had no mother to love and care for him, it was best that he had been taken.

While the Yoders and I were at dinner the next day, we heard the unmistakable sound of *xich-lo* bells. The bells seemed louder than usual; it was Sunday, early in the afternoon, and there was no other traffic on our road. Dr. Yoder and I went out and found two children being carried from the *xich-lo* by their father. The man said he was Nam's brother-in-law. He thought the children were sick with the same thing as his small son, who had died the night before.

The youngsters, a girl of four and a boy of thirteen, were placed in the doctor's offce to keep contamination at a minimum and we went to work on them immediately. Fortunately, though they were in great pain, the lymph gland enlargement was confined mainly to their armpits. Their symptoms were milder than their brother's had been, and we started oral doses of sulfa drugs and streptomycin injections.

While I stayed with them, Dr. Yoder left the Chan-Y-Vien on his regular visit to the Eighth Field Hospital, to check on some laboratory results. He spoke with the physicians there, describing the symptoms of the three children. They mentioned various kinds of lymphatic infection and then Dr. Tsang said, "Have you thought of plague?"

He had heard of a few cases of bubonic plague up near Hue, although none had been reported yet in our area. Dr. Yoder hurried back, stopping only at the Province Hospital to alert the staff there to the possibility that we had had a plague death and were treating two other cases.

When Dr. Yoder returned and told us of the probable diagnosis, we discussed the likelihood of a widespread outbreak. We tried to account for the severity of the youngest child's illness in comparison with that of his brother and sister. We decided that, because he had been so young, he had not been able to communicate the fact that he was in pain until it was too late and the infection had progressed too far. The pain from the swelling in the lymph nodes is the first and most recognizable symptom of bubonic plague. Also, because he had been younger he had less resistance to infection generally than the other two and therefore developed a more severe infection more rapidly. In addition, the father was by now alerted to the presence of illness in his family and was looking for symptoms. Fortunately the two older children seemed to be responding well to the medication.

We did not have to wait long to have our fears of a rising incidence of bubonic plague in our area confirmed. By the time these two children were out of danger, several other cases had been reported. Within a week, bubonic plague was showing up in widely divergent sections of Nhatrang. With the sudden rise in the dreaded sickness, there was tremendous concern and fear both on the part of the authorities and the public. Work to exterminate rats—which carry the plague-transmitting flea—from all districts where plague victims lived was begun. Anti-plague inoculation centers were set up throughout the city with speed and efficiency that were little short of miraculous for Vietnam.

Our part in the program was to inoculate the 350 children at the orphanage next door, and see that the 100 students at the nearby Bible School also had shots. The serum was provided by the local health authorities through the Institute Pasteur. The Army provided us with quantities of disposable hypodermic needles.

The orphans were to come first. Very early in the morning we watched them as they walked single file, the smallest one in front, along the beach and then onto our road. When they reached the hospital, we divided them into four groups. Dr. Yoder, Phyllis, Anh Tin, and I had the necessary supplies on a table. A group lined up in front of each of us. We injected several of the older children first and then had them stand by as helpers, wiping the arm of a waiting child with alcohol before the injection and wiping it again after the needle was withdrawn.

The children offered no resistance—and almost no tears. As soon as his inoculation was over, each ran back to the orphanage. All were taken care of in about two hours.

The delegation from the Bible School, all of them eighteen years or older, took their injections with far less aplomb than the youngsters. Though there were only a third as many, the students kept us busy for almost the same length of time.

The Chan-Y-Vien received no more bubonic plague patients after that, and in a short while—thanks to mass inoculations throughout the area and the program of rat extermination—Nhatrang did not have to contend with any more plague cases.

However, the fear and excitement of the plague scare had

no sooner died down than our province was shocked by an incident of a different kind. It followed a pattern of Buddhist protests against the government that had been recurring sporadically ever since the shooting of eight Buddhists during the uprising in Hue in May. In June an aged monk had set fire to himself and in the next few months several others did likewise. But our area had remained untouched by this religio-political conflict. Now we heard that a young Buddhist nun in Nhatrang had attempted to burn herself alive. The local police, alerted to her intention, were standing by and immediately threw water on her flaming robes. She suffered only slight burns as a result.

As a penalty for her actions, the nun was deported to her family's village, about 19 miles from Nhatrang. There the unfortunate and perhaps demented young woman again doused herself with gasoline and was consumed by flames.

The suicidal act was horrible and, to Westerners, was an incomprehensible way of making a political protest. We discussed the possible repercussions in Nhatrang, wondering if there would be more self-immolations. While no more local Buddhists set fire to themselves, other such incidents continued to occur in Saigon and Hue. We speculated on the psychology of those who chose self-immolation as a means of protest. The case of the young girl was even harder to comprehend than the death of the monks. Then we heard rumors about the girl. One story was that she was not a nun at all, but a seventeen-year-old who had become pregnant out of wedlock. By the time I left Nhatrang two years later, she would be immortalized. There would be a bust of her in the park near the post office where she first tried to burn herself. The park itself would become a sort of memorial, containing plaques showing the flame and the lotus flower—the symbol of Buddhism.

As far as Nhatrang was concerned, calm was restored and life went on as usual. We at the Chan-Y-Vien, with a continuing increase in patients, concentrated on our work. The restrictions of the fortified hamlet program had long been forgotten—the gates were left open at all hours and no alarms broke the stillness of the nights.

In October an Air Force captain stationed in Nhatrang was reported missing in action over North Vietnam. He was flying a photo reconnaissance mission and failed to return. I knew the young captain well. Only the week before I had met him and we had stopped to chat over a cup of coffee. He was ecstatically happy over a picture he had just received of his infant daughter. He had never seen the child, who was born after he went overseas. At the time we ran into each other he had less than a month of his Vietnam tour left to serve. He was literally counting the hours until he would be reunited with his wife and baby.

There was no way of knowing the fate of the captain, but his chances of remaining alive were considered slim. His fate made the war seem more senseless to all of us than ever.

During the last week in October the political situation in Saigon came suddenly and explosively to a head. I first heard the news from Anh Tin at the hospital. During his evening duty Anh Tin usually kept his radio going; it was during one of his listening periods that a Vietnamese news broadcast hinted that all was not well in the capital. All day vague rumors of trouble were murmured around the hospital by other workers. What was happening was still unclear, but the Vietnamese knew, in spite of government censorship of the news, that trouble was brewing or had already arrived. Dr. Yoder, Phyllis, and I were too busy to take time out and listen to the daytime Armed Forces Radio broadcasts from

Saigon. And we knew that, because of the censorship, few facts would be made immediately available anyway.

At dinner time the three of us gathered around the Yoders' shortwave set—only to hear news about everything except what was happening in Saigon. The next night it was different; the first report we heard was that President Ngo Dinh Diem and his brother Ngo Dinh Nhu had been deposed by a military coup. A few hours later, a Voice of America broadcast from Manila announced that both the brothers had been assassinated. The detested Madame Nhu, who had been such a power in her brother-in-law's government, was reportedly on her way to the United States.

The plot and all its ramifications were revealed gradually over the next few days. From what I could gather, Diem's brother had indicated a willingness to negotiate with the Vietcong to end the war. This, apparently, was the immediate cause of the coup. But it had been coming for some time and much broader grievances were at its root.

There was little reliable information in our area about the man who replaced Diem, Duong Van Minh. It was clear that he was supported by the United States, but less clear what his position was among his countrymen. But Minh's regime would be shortlived, as would his successor's. Until there could be a free election, there seemed to be little hope for political stability.

Madame Nhu, disliked as she was, spent the next weeks and months rallying support for her cause in the West. It was generally accepted in Vietnam that the source of her wealth was misappropriated American aid. All of us felt that the country was well rid of her. The next week, during a short vacation at Dalat, I saw her famous summer villa, a sumptuous white palace set at the top of a series of mountain terraces. While her people were deprived of so many of life's essentials and her country was at war, Madame Nhu had had this lavish retreat built, no expense spared, as a private hideaway. Now, only a few days after her husband's assassination, it stood deserted and empty, a symbol of the futility of corrupted power.

While a new government was taking over in Saigon, civilian air transportation was banned—but that interruption of service lasted only a few days. Otherwise nothing seemed to have been disturbed. As far as we could judge from observing the behavior of people in Nhatrang, everything was as usual.

18

In november the rainy season began. Hai and I could no longer go for daybreak walks along the beach and hunt for shells. Always an early riser, I found this the best time of day for enjoying the beauty of the sea and the sand.

One morning in the middle of the month when it was raining most heavily and I was alone in the kitchen making a pot of before-breakfast coffee, the hospital's night worker came to the back door. As usual he spoke very rapidly and it took a few minutes for me to grasp what he was trying to tell me. A very sick woman, he said, was on the front verandah of the hospital with her brother. They had told the worker they would sit by the door until clinic opened. But when he heard her severe cough and noted how very thin and frail she was, he thought we ought to be notified. I thanked him and told him to go back and say I would be over immediately to see them.

The woman was in her early sixties, wrinkled, with sparse gray hair pinned in a small tight knot at the back of her head. She was emaciated to the point of skin and bones. She and her brother, whom I recognized as living in the neighborhood, told me about her medical background. She had a long history of irregular treatment for tuberculosis, and severe episodes of hemorrhage. She was well-to-do and had been well cared for by local standards. Nevertheless, the disease had progressed to the point where it had done irreparable damage to her health.

Not everyone who came to the Chan-Y-Vien was poor. Rich people came too, brought by its reputation for good treatment. First, probably, they would have shopped around among the physicians in private practice in Nhatrang, of whom there were quite a few even though most of the Vietnamese doctors at this time were in the army. They were French-trained, but they lacked the hospital experience that American doctors are required to have before entering practice.

There was no doubt that this woman was critically ill. After Dr. Yoder examined her we put her in the small three-bed isolated room just off the ward. She was attended by a woman servant, hired by the brother. The maid never left her mistress, sleeping at night in a canvas deck chair by her bedside.

The sick woman was a devout Buddhist. She kept her prayer beads in her hands and was constantly saying her devotions. Another brother, a Buddhist monk, clad in a gray robe, came to visit several times. He belonged to a worldly order that moved freely among people. The monks in saffron yellow, whom we saw more frequently, had taken vows of poverty, renouncing all material things, and when they went into public places kept their heads down and spoke only when it was absolutely necessary.

While the Vietnamese maid was tireless in making the elderly lady comfortable, I could not induce her to give her mistress daily sponge baths. By this time I was not surprised. Only the most educated of the Vietnamese have accepted the standards of personal hygiene known in the West. At first this disregard for personal cleanliness aroused my crusading instinct. With the outpatients my advice fell on deaf ears. With ward patients, however, we had to be insistent about bathing. But the kind of cleanliness that's routine in American hospitals could never be maintained.

Our Vietnamese aides so completely identified with the attitude of the patients that they could not be relied on to give bed baths. And so I had to do it. When a new patient was required to submit to a sponging, the others would sympathize in good humor with his discomfort while assuring him that the soap and water wouldn't attract evil spirits. Hardest to convince of the necessity for cleanliness were the mothers with babies and small children, who of course needed it most. They were particularly fearful of calling the attention of the spirits to their offspring.

The Vietnamese are extremely concerned about spirits. There were several times when Hai came to me frightened, after hearing strange noises in the night, convinced that there were ghosts wandering about. Even a fair number of Vietnamese Christians have a fear of spirits, retaining some traces of the superstitions of the primitive animistic religion that was native to their land before either Buddhism or Christianity arrived.

The Land-Rover had long been ready for the junk heap. We never knew from one day to the next whether its motor would start up, and flat tires had become so common that we all became expert at changing them in near record time. But the fund-raising campaign to buy us a Volkswagen pickup had not yet reached its quota. Army personnel from the Nhatrang area would come upon one of us stuck in the middle of the road so frequently that they decided interim measures had to be taken.

On one of the rare sunny afternoons we had that November, I went down to the beach with Hai for a swim. We were returning to the bungalow when we were greeted by a master sergeant and an enlisted man—friends of ours and the hospital. They had just emerged from a towering, massive two-and-a-half-ton military truck. That is, it had once been a military truck, but it had shed its previous coat of olive drab and was now painted the most outrageous shade of robin's egg blue imaginable.

The sergeant, ignoring my dripping wet bathing suit, made a speech. "With our compliments and best wishes," he announced with all the solemnity he could muster, nodding toward the truck, "we have brought you 'The Blue Goose' for the hospital; use and enjoy it until your Volkswagen arrives. We have chosen the color with great care," he added, "to match your eyes. We hope it suits you."

His short speech had ended. I stood there dumbfounded, not daring to take another look at the behemoth that loomed before me. Then the pretense of solemnity gave way and we all burst out laughing. The sergeant led me over to examine the gift, but we were laughing so hard now that it took several attempts to boost me up into the eight-foot-high cab of the truck. And, once inside, the absurdity of me in my wet suit sitting behind the steering wheel sent me into another paroxysm of giggles.

Leave it to the Army to think big! It didn't occur to me to

ask about the source of the gift, but it was probable that a high-ranking officer would have had to approve the truck's "diversion" to us before we could have received it.

Once I was behind the wheel, the soldiers wanted me to try it out—for size, as they put it. There was nothing I wanted to do less than maneuver the cavernous vehicle, but I had no choice. Gingerly I started up the motor with the sergeant directing as I manipulated. The sound that emerged was agonizing and almost paralyzed me with fear. But I went on, afraid that if I gave up now I'd never again get behind the wheel. I had to use both hands to shift. And if I failed to remember the double clutching it could have been disastrous.

Slowly I inched the Blue Goose down the path to the road. Once it got going, it handled much more easily than I had expected. But I couldn't judge its size and was certain I'd never be able to back it up, or get it through the gate and onto the road in one maneuver.

I drove for a mile or so along the road past the hospital and turned out onto the main road. Then I turned back. Children from the orphanage and then those that lived in the neighborhood came running out to watch us lumbering by. I began to feel like the Pied Piper, for they all fell into line behind us, running and laughing as the monster headed back to the Chan-Y-Vien. By the time I brought the truck to a halt I think that just about every child and adult in the vicinity had assembled. When we dismounted they began scrambling over the vehicle and clambering aboard via a yellow ladder in the rear.

The Yoders came out to see what was going on, and by now the front yard looked as though a spontaneous celebration was taking place. Their own reaction was identical to mine when they saw the "Goose." They doubled over with laughter and we all joined in with them again. It was one of the gayest times ever spent at the Chan-Y-Vien. But it was the last time any of us would feel like laughing for many weeks to come.

I remember Saturday morning was gray and rainy. As soon as breakfast was finished I went to the hospital to make preparations for the eye surgery that would be performed later by Dr. Yoder and one of the Army doctors. Suddenly Phyllis came flying in.

"President Kennedy has been assassinated—he was shot and killed!"

Her voice was strong with emotion. Her eyes were bright with tears.

"It can't be—that's impossible," I said.

"No—no—it's true—one of the missionary wives from the hill heard it on an early Voice of America broadcast—she came and told us."

I still felt the news had been misunderstood; the President might have been shot, but surely he wasn't dead.

Phyllis and I went back to the bungalow and sat with Dr. Yoder, listening to the fateful and all too true news being broadcast by Armed Forces Radio in Saigon.

When the Army surgeon arrived, he and Dr. Yoder agreed that the eye operations should be postponed for several days. Of course the regular routine could not come to a halt, so after the Army surgeon left, Dr. Yoder and I went to the hospital and checked the ward patients. Since it was Saturday there would be no clinic and our work would be minimal. Then, shaken, we returned to stay all day by the radio.

The shock, the unbelievable horror with which we reacted to the President's assassination was too deep to describe.

Our reaction was no different from that of people all over the world—disbelief followed by a feeling of intense personal loss. We could have felt no greater grief had we learned of a death in each of our own families.

From the Voice of America and the Armed Forces Radio Station in Saigon we heard of the circumstances of the President's murder. Although it was Saturday in Nhatrang, because of the time differential it was still that fateful Friday in Dallas. Very gradually we began to accept the reality of what had occurred. We heard a recording of Lyndon B. Johnson taking the oath of office as President and, shortly afterward, the news that the assassin had himself been killed. It couldn't have been long after we first received word of President Kennedy's death when Vietnamese friends began to convey their condolences to us.

The reactions were rather amazing under the political circumstances that existed at that time. From the well-educated social elite down to the illiterate peasants there was genuine sympathy. I'm certain that many of the people who expressed their sorrow knew virtually nothing about John Kennedy beyond his name. But they did know how highly esteemed he was by his countrymen. And among those who knew more about him, people with access to newspapers and radio, there was a personally felt respect. Anh Tin summed up the feeling among the Vietnamese when he told me, "You have lost a dear and honored leader. We are truly sorry."

In the next weeks one of my main sources of information about what was happening in the States was my family, which sent me letters and clippings from the American press, including speculations about changes in policy that might take place now that Mr. Johnson was President.

Shortly after Tet of 1964 the Minh government fell and Major General Nguyen Khanh succeeded him as president.

American recognition of Khanh came soon afterward, based largely on the recommendation of the new American ambassador, General Maxwell Taylor, who had replaced Ambassador Henry Cabot Lodge. With this recognition it seemed likely that there would be few immediate changes in American policy.

19

AFTER THE NEW YEAR, the Yoders and I agreed that Hai no longer required hospitalization and constant medical supervision.

By Vietnamese standards he had become a spoiled and lazy child, although by our standards he was an ordinary little boy. Had he been living with a Vietnamese family, his life would have been far different. Since there are usually many children in a family and since they are born in rapid succession, barring miscarriage, they are expected at a very early age to take on household responsibilities. As soon as an infant reaches the toddling stage he is given such chores as watching his younger baby brother or sister. When a new child is born into the family, the older ones become responsible for him. There is little time to play, and toys and games as we know them simply don't exist. By the time a child is ten he is expected to assume whatever duties his family assigns him.

Even though Hai had a married sister who, now that he was well, would welcome him into her home, we felt a degree of responsibility for seeing that his bright young mind received formal schooling.

Dr. Yoder, who took care of all the Foster Parent Plan families in our province, decided to find out whether Hai's family was eligible for inclusion in this program. The Foster Parent Plan operates throughout the world. Its purpose is to see that needy families with school-age children are given monetary support, provided that these children are kept in school.

After a Vietnamese social worker associated with the F.P.P. certified that Hai's family was eligible, it was arranged to send him to his sister's home. Since she lived in our area, Hai would be able to return to the Chan-Y-Vien at regular intervals for a clinic checkup, so we would not sever all relations with him.

Hai said he was glad that he would be going to school, that it was the hope of every Vietnamese to become educated, and that he would show his gratitude by studying hard, hoping some day to be able to pass the entrance examination for the university.

For a going-away gift, Phyllis and I bought Hai new clothes and some school supplies. One day not long after he left the hospital we passed him on the road near his village. He was in the company of some schoolmates and he seemed as happy as we had ever seen him.

The Chan-Y-Vien facilities were often sorely tried. There simply weren't enough hands or equipment for all that had to be done. Construction of a new wing had been begun, as

Rudi Lichti had promised, but we were still handling a vastly increased patient load with the same small overworked staff. Our activities made such a small dent in the multitude of medical problems existing around us that it sometimes seemed utterly futile. The average Vietnamese life span was thirty-two years. And the main causes of death remained malnutrition and tuberculosis. It was impossible to see how this situation could be changed until the Vietnamese government set up public health clinics in every large community. But the war made such a program virtually impossible. Funds were insufficient, there was no equipment, and the necessary personnel was not available.

In the late winter of 1964 there was another outbreak of cholera. Fortunately, prompt distribution of serum and wholesale inoculation of the populace contained it before it got out of hand. With adequate medical supplies, and thanks to our previous experience, lives were saved.

But the number of patients we lost was still too great. People came to us when it was too late for us to help them. The most heartbreaking of these were patients with advanced tuberculosis. The pulmonary infection is the aspect of the disease that is most familiar. But in addition, it attacks the bones and skin, making rapid inroads which are frightful to see and agonizing for the victims.

One pathetic case was that of little San. Only four months old, he had already contracted a severe case of tuberculosis of the skin. There was a breakdown of skin behind one ear and on part of his scalp. Necrosis and sloughing off of the tissue had already set in when we saw him. Long-term care, which included much medication and daily changes of the dressings over the afflicted areas, resulted in the child's eventual recovery. Only a small scar remained as a reminder of his severe illness. As long as medication was continued after his discharge from the hospital and as long as he received regular check-ups, it was likely that there would be no recurrence. We could only hope that San's mother would not think her child cured for all time and fail to see that he received continuing treatment.

But unfortunately not all cases had happy endings. I recall a one-year-old boy suffering from a bilateral pulmonary infection. In spite of intensive treatment, his disease, too far advanced when he came to us, was fatal.

Saddest of all tubercular cases was when a mother and child, or a whole family, was infected. It was not uncommon for us to care for entire families in the annex and, later, in the new barracks built especially for the tuberculosis patients behind the hospital.

I came to regard tuberculosis as the most detestable of all diseases that take human life. Once it gains a firm foothold in a person, it marches on, often defying all medicine. The tragedy was that we saw so many of these cases when it was too late. I have lost count of the times I stood helplessly at a bedside, knowing there was nothing that could be done to keep that patient alive.

In Vietnam many teenagers were struck down by the disease. We could not let them know that they would never reach adulthood. We would talk to them about the future, giving them courage for the little time that remained. For an older advanced case, such as the wealthy Buddhist lady who was then with us, there was little we could do except make the patient as comfortable as possible. Medication—isoniazid, streptomycin, and para-amino-salicylic acid—could prolong life somewhat, but one could not even hope for a cure for most of our tuberculosis patients.

One stormy spring night I was awakened by the aide on duty at the hospital. He was standing outside my window and calling to me. The wind and the rain that night were so violent that I could barely make out his face through the space between the louvers and I was unable to hear what he was saying. But I knew that, if he had subjected himself to the driving rain, there must be an emergency in the ward.

I dressed quickly and raced through the downpour into the rear entrance of the hospital. All the lights were on in the ward and the patients were all wide awake, but quiet. In the silence I could hear the elderly lady in isolation coughing violently. Her frightened maid stood in the doorway. She said she had been doing her best to help, but had not been able to stop the lady's coughing which, I could see, by now had induced hemorrhaging.

Minutes after my arrival the patient collapsed and died. I sent the maid to notify the family. While she was gone I cleaned up as much as possible the visible signs of the poor woman's violent end that were on her clothing and the bed. Then I covered her body with a sheet.

By the time the woman's brother arrived, his sister's body had been moved into the operating room, which was usually used as a temporary morgue. He and the maid set out candles and incense on a low stool that was nearby. At daybreak the brother who was a monk came, and from then on there was a constant procession of mourners coming and going during the early morning. Luckily, due to the heavy rain, there was only light attendance at clinic. After several other monks arrived, a funeral service was begun. Our outpatients, with natural curiosity, were loath to leave.

My curiosity, too, was aroused. Since the woman was a Buddhist, we had expected that she would be taken home just before death came. But it had come suddenly. It had never occurred to us that the elaborate ceremony due one of her devoutness and position might take place at the Chan-Y-Vien.

The chanting of an ancient prayer for the dead went on

and on. The sound of a gourd rattle being shaken underscored the eerie tonal rise and fall of the incantation. We could easily have been hypnotized by the sound. Every so often one of the three bonzes—as the monks are called—would leave the operating room and go out and peer down the lane. They took turns doing this most of the morning.

Toward noon a black panel truck drove up to the hospital. The lookout monk returned to the operating room and the chanting ceased. Men got out of the truck and brought a coffin up onto the verandah. One of the monks, standing in the doorway of the operating room, told them to enter. The coffin bearers came out emptyhanded and returned to their truck. I was startled to see the driver start up the engine and drive off. Dr. Yoder and I had fully expected that the dead woman would be put in the coffin and taken away in the truck. But apparently the religious ceremony would go on.

For a while there was silence from the operating room. But while I was making a quick round of the ward, finding all the patients quiet despite their curiosity, the chanting was resumed. This time it was accompanied by the slow sounding of a gong as well as the rattling gourds. Both doors to the operating room were open. I looked in and saw that the coffin was open, with lighted candles standing at the head and foot. Clusters of lighted joss sticks were emitting a heavy perfumed smoke.

On and on went the ceremony. The monks, seated cross-legged on the floor in the lotus position, never stopped chanting. The steady stream of visitors continued. The family members, in white, were easy to identify. Friends of the dead woman's relatives, including several gray-robed Buddhist nuns, swelled the group of mourners. By now the clinic room and the verandah were crowded with people. And *xichlos*, automobiles, buses, and motor scooters filled our road.

182

Dr. Yoder and I did not need to make ourselves unobtrusive—nobody paid any attention to us. We had several severely ill patients in the ward, and neither the activity in and around the hospital nor the knowledge that a funeral was in progress was conducive to their rest. Yet to request that the funeral rite be hurried seemed inappropriate.

Later in the afternoon, traffic in the road pulled over to make way for a black hearse. The family in the operating room was notified. The chanting ceased. The red lid was put on the coffin and the candles were transferred to the top. The monks left the room first, going out of the building and into waiting *xich-los.* Then the procession formed behind them. Black-robed pallbearers placed the coffin in the hearse. Slowly, accompanied by the booming of the gong, the procession moved down the road. Bits of paper, symbolizing money, were strewn by members of the family to insure that the spirit of the departed would have sufficient funds for the journey to heaven.

It was more than twelve hours since the elderly woman had died. During that whole time it had been impossible to maintain the normal hospital routine. After it was all over we could only hope that it would never become necessary for another Buddhist funeral to be held on the premises.

Cleaning up the operating room, I could still smell the heavy fragrance of the incense. It hung in the air for another day and served as a reminder of the strange scene we had witnessed.

20

Our volkswagen pickup finally arrived one day, driven by a small delegation of G.I.s. It was well worth waiting for. What a pleasure it was to step into the blue cab after the climbing we had had to do in order to drive our previous conveyances! A curved metal roof lined with pasteboard protected the back and its passengers from the heat and sun, and when the tailgate was down, one big hop or step up was all that was needed to climb aboard. Although its arrival was not accompanied by the carnival atmosphere that had greeted the Blue Goose, we were delighted with the new vehicle.

The Yoders had still not found the child they wanted. They were looking for a part-Vietnamese, part-American child, of which there now were an increasing number. But not all such children were available for adoption. One of the Chan-Y-Vien's directors suggested that they try Saigon, where there were several Protestant orphanages, and they planned to spend a few days there. The night before they left we had a gala dinner together and I wished them the best in finding the daughter they wanted.

But they returned from Saigon without a child, thinking they would have to abandon the idea entirely.

Phyllis threw herself more deeply into her work than ever before and the doctor and she rarely left the hospital. It wasn't difficult to become completely occupied with matters at the Chan-Y-Vien since the workload had by now become staggering. Although it was late summer, and the weather was stiflingly hot, attendance at clinic continued to mount. Clinic hours had to be extended to one in the afternoon and there were days when we still couldn't accommodate all who came. Patients would line up on the verandah as early as five in the morning and by seven there were usually more than two hundred, with more arriving later. Many of these people had traveled most of the previous day to come for treatment. Those who arrived too late for one clinic session, or who needed to remain for daily treatment and lived too far away to return home and come back in one day, slept on mats on the floor of the verandah or in hammocks slung between the trees, despite the mosquitoes and in defiance of the night air, something they usually dreaded.

We always had mosquitoes and flies in abundance. Screens had been put in the windows of the hospital but the patients would swing them open in order to get a clearer view of whatever might be going on outside, and the flies and other insects entered the ward without hindrance. I would give the patients rolled-up newspapers and tell them to swat the flies; at one time I even offered a reward—one piaster for every fifteen dead flies.

The crowd that was now almost constantly on the premises compounded another problem that we always faced—

wads of chewed betel nut all over the ground. The women chewed constantly and expectorated everywhere. Ba'-Ba was constantly picking up the little wads, but there would be another collection by the time she had finished. Finally we decided to make spittoons available. We bought a quantity of inexpensive metal chamber pots and tied them to trees around the Chan-Y-Vien. But it seemed that the women would go out of their way to spit everywhere but in the new spittoons, and we just gave up.

We had hoped that the new wing would be finished by this time, but work still remained to be done on it. We had said goodbye to Rudi and Elda Lichti at the beginning of the summer and had greeted their successors, Paul and Doris Longacre. The Longacres were a young couple, still in their early twenties, who had elected to spend three years in service with the Mennonite Central Committee after Paul's graduation from Goshen Seminary. They would supervise the M.C.C.'s food distribution program, try to recruit replacement and additional staff members for us, and act as business managers and liaison agents for us in Saigon.

As yet there was no word about receiving another M.C.C. nurse to assist us. Our Vietnamese staff consisted of three girls to help with nursing and clinic chores and three young men who helped the doctor in the clinic and also in the ward. The girls, when they first came to us, were usually untrained, and their skills were sorely inadequate. We had to teach them the very basics of the profession, beginning with taking a patient's temperature. They were eager and quick to learn, in spite of the language barrier which made teaching so difficult. With the aid of an interpreter, Phyllis gave the workers classes in basic nursing skills and pharmacology. Dr. Yoder expanded their abilities by lecturing on the diseases and health problems they would be encountering while working with us.

Later, our staff was augmented by several girls
taken various nursing courses then being offered in
These training programs lasted from six months to
years, but even this background was inadequate preparat
for the demands that would be placed on them at the Chan
Y-Vien. Nevertheless, with time and effort on our part, we
were able to develop several invaluable aides. Anh Tin, one
of our best, was still with us, now promoted to being Dr. Yoder's surgical assistant. Dr. Yoder had begun gradually to allow
him to do more and more of each entropion procedure under
his guidance until Anh Tin was now capable of repairing
eyelids without supervision. His pride in his work and accomplishment was a real pleasure to all of us.

One of the most agreeable and competent of the girls was
Co Trang. She was a Buddhist, the only non-Christian member of the staff who was to remain permanently. She had
been with us for several months when we found out one day
that she had been dismissed by our directors.

Some valuable and potent drugs had mysteriously disappeared, and the disappearance was finally traced to another
Buddhist girl who was working as our laboratory technician.
Because of this unfortunate incident, the girl was asked by
the Board to leave, and because Co Trang was a friend of
hers and had been hired on the technician's recommendation, she was also asked to leave. In notifying us of its decision, the Board said that only Christian personnel should be
hired for work in the Chan-Y-Vien in the future. We and the
staff who worked with Co Trang were furious, for her quiet
way with the patients and her good working relationship
with her Vietnamese colleagues had endeared her to all.

After a few weeks, Dr. Yoder learned that Co Trang
would be willing to let bygones be bygones, and on his own
authority asked her to return to work with us. He quietly
explained to the Board that with the increased work load we

ʜer capabilities. He also reminded them
ɴation was un-Christian and that we
ᴅless of religion. He argued that this
ᴏ the staff as well. So the matter was

ᴛ time to myself, I rarely went into
ᴘɪᴄᴋ up the mail and make hospital pur-
ᴏn sunny weekends I tried to find a few hours to get
ᴅᴏwn to the cove to swim and luxuriate in its quiet. But this
peace was increasingly shattered by planes flying overhead.
Enormous jets, troop and cargo carriers, teams of helicopters, and small reconnaissance planes came and went from
the airport almost without let-up.

The number of aircraft was drastically increased in the
early fall. North Vietnamese torpedo boats had attacked two
U.S. destroyers in the Bay of Tonkin in August. Until then
there had been no direct confrontation between the United
States and North Vietnam. But now President Johnson
ordered retaliatory action. And so the worst was begun.

It was impossible to close our eyes to what was happening. If we could forget for a few moments that American
soldiers were being wounded and killed, we would be
quickly reminded when an American jet streaked over the
Chan-Y-Vien. And the mounting number of casualties at the
Eighth Field Hospital would continue to attest to the fact
that the United States was now inextricably involved in
combat in South Vietnam.

But aside from the increased evidence of American military participation, we were untouched by the heightened
conflict. Life went on for us pretty much as it had before and
even social activities were undisturbed.

To fulfill some of the social obligations that I had in-
curred, I decided to invite several of my friends, all of whom

were involved in our work, to dinner. A Vietnamese husband and wife dining out together in public is not uncommon but for these friends it was a luxury. When I extended an invitation to three couples who lived nearby, they accepted with pleasure and excitement.

We were to be a party of seven. But at the last minute I decided to bring along a thirteen-year-old boy, who was one of our patients at the time, as my escort. Diep was an orphan who had had most of the bones of one leg destroyed by tubercular osteomyelitis. He had become very attached to the Yoders and me and we often included him in our plans.

Before we went to dinner I took my guests for a drive along the beautiful Beach Highway. Strangely, although they had lived in Nhatrang all their lives, not all of them had ever been this far from town. They marveled at the beauty of the sea and hills as if they were seeing their country for the first time. It was likely that this would be as much of their country as they would ever see; people in the provincial cities rarely had cause or enough money to travel any distance from home, and now that road travel was becoming increasingly difficult and in some places impossible, it was not likely that their mobility would be improved.

For dinner we went to a restaurant famous for *pho*, pronounced "fa," which was a dish of noodles, meat, bean sprouts and consommé, topped with the ever-present *nuoc mam*. The restaurant's tiny kitchen opened onto the street and we passed it before we entered. As we went by, the men called out our order to the cook. Then we sat down and, ignoring the other patrons' curious stares, threw ourselves wholeheartedly into the business of eating. We had decided we would make dinner a contest of sorts, the object being to see who could consume the most bowls of *pho*. Laughing and making jokes, the men proceeded to eat several each, compared with the modest two bowls for each of the ladies. Diep won after emptying four bowls and then almost falling asleep.

Our party went on long after we finished dinner. The Vietnamese laugh and talk very easily. If I had been regarded as a stranger, the evening could have been a serious, formal event with conversation limited to only the most polite small talk, but since these were people I knew well and worked with, we thoroughly enjoyed ourselves.

After dinner we browsed in several of the nearby shops and each of the women bought me a little figure carved from a piece of shell. Because they were my friends they would not leave me without giving me a token gift. To my protests they rejoined that they enjoyed giving something that they themselves would like to have.

Our friends and patients were often so generous that it was embarrassing and overwhelming. Flowers, eggs, fruit, ducks, and chickens, as well as more expensive and exotic gifts, were heaped on us. The father of one of our patients— a little boy who had been critically ill with a kidney infection—presented Dr. Yoder with a peacock. He apologized for giving only one, explaining that he had bought two, but the other had sickened and died. The cost of peacocks was extremely high by local standards, the equivalent of eight American dollars, and its giver was a man of modest circumstances at best. So the peacock took up residence with the dogs, and various other animals in the garden, adding his beautiful colors to our small menagerie.

A few weeks later a convoy of U.S. Navy destroyers and corvettes arrived, reportedly on a training mission, and anchored in the Nhatrang harbor. For the week they were there it looked like a carnival at sea. High-ranking Vietnamese men and their wives were invited aboard at various times to observe the ships and visit with the crews. A nearby hill overlooked the city and harbor, and from the top of it we could see the ships as clearly as if they were moored in the cove. At night the lights strung from their masts and outlining their hulls transformed the harbor into a scene from a fairy tale. All of Nhatrang went down to the beach to see the lovely sight. Only a little persuasion was necessary to talk me into loading the Volkswagen with patients and neighborhood children. Off we drove for a closer look at the wondrous sight of the American ships. When I explained to my wide-eyed truckload that these were ships sent by my country, they thought me very lucky to belong to a nation that had such beautiful vessels in its navy. They were incredulous when I told them that in the United States there were even much larger ships, that could carry hundreds of people across huge expanses of water with all the comforts and conveniences of our homes. For these people knew only the small freighters which transported goods from Saigon, and the small wooden or woven bamboo boats with which their fishermen braved the seas.

While the ships were still in Nhatrang harbor, a Vietcong battalion blew up a train about 12 miles to the west of us. Several Vietnamese were killed and many more were injured. We feared this would affect people's methods of transportation to and from the hospital. But apparently the local people thought otherwise, for there was no indication that the patients coming to the clinic were greatly disturbed by the incident. Nighttime travel had long ago been limited because of bad roads, curtailed bus schedules, and the curfew, but travel during the day was much the same as always. Gradually, however, the number of miles that people could travel by bus was reduced, due to the bombing and blasting of roads and bridges. But still the patients continued to arrive, even from the areas where several hamlets were under rebel control.

After the Yoders returned from a week's missionary conference, they told me they had decided that I should take a short rest and that they were treating me to a weekend at Dalat. The place we always stayed at in the cool mountain city was a guest house run by the Overseas Crusade missionaries. It was a lovely place set in the midst of a pine forest. The charmingly furnished rooms and the large open fireplace in the main living-dining room made one feel comfortably at home.

Although I had no plans except to relax, I was delighted to accept an invitation from the missionary couple who maintained the guest house to join them in an overnight trip. They were going to a Koho tribal village in the nearby Dran valley and the excursion would combine missionary work with hunting. Two other workers would be joining them, all teaching missionaries. Because they had been working with the Koho tribes for some time, they knew the people and the language well. When I climbed into the Land-Rover I saw that it was solidly packed with equipment. I caught a glimpse of a collapsible cot under a tarpaulin, along with cooking utensils and much safari equipment. My host was well known by the tribespeople as well as by other missionaries as a good and keen hunter, an accomplishment highly esteemed by the Kohos.

After a three-hour hair-raising drive over narrow mountain roads and then a bumpy ride over roads rutted and laced with small crude wooden bridges in the valley itself, we arrived at our destination, Sa May, one of several small Koho villages scattered throughout the valley. We drove through the gate and into the hamlet, stopping beside a house that looked newer than its neighbors. Immediately we

192

were surrounded by villagers who welcomed us graciously and enthusiastically. They set to work unloading the truck for us and I was amazed to see enough paraphernalia emerge to set up permanent housekeeping. There were beds, sleeping bags, and pillows; a number of cartons containing cutlery, pots, pans, and canned food, as well as the powerful searchlights, guns, and boxes of shells brought for the safari. The latter items were, of course, the main objects of interest to those helping to unload. Last to be removed was a simple slide projector and a box of slides. The heavy generator that would provide the electric power to run the projector was left in the Rover, along with yards and yards of heavy electrical cord.

I couldn't help comparing all these supplies with the way the Chan-Y-Vien's Land-Rover had so often been packed for its expeditions to tribal villages. It too was filled to capacity with vast amounts of equipment, but of a very different kind.

We had been given the best house in the village, the home of the tribe's pastor, while he and his family moved temporarily into the home of a parishioner. Everything was done to make us comfortable. While some villagers set up our camp beds, others came with hot water so that we might wash away the grime of the journey. Still others brought steaming hot tea and fruit. At lunch, which included both Western-style food, which we had brought, and dishes prepared by the villagers, we were joined by the pastor and two other men from the community. Afterward we went on a short tour of the village. The interiors of the homes were bare and simple and filled with smoke from the open fireplaces. Most contained little furniture except for a crude bed and perhaps one or two stools. The pastor, himself a tribesman, served as our guide and interpreter.

When the people learned that I was a nurse there were

special requests that I visit homes where a member of a family was ill. Not having brought medicines with me, I could only provide some simple common-sense advice. I gave instructions for washing and dressing wounds caused by the pungi stakes placed in the jungle around the village to keep out marauders. I gave diet instructions for patients with ulcer symptoms, and one small child with a high temperature was sponged with tepid water until he rested more comfortably. The tribespeople were simple, friendly, and trusting, as had been those I had worked with in the Nhatrang area. Many of them were in poor health. I was told that the nearest hospital was a considerable distance away and while the local missionaries distributed simple remedies, the serious cases generally had to go untreated.

The event for which we had come took place after dinner that night in front of the framework of a large new wooden church being built by the villagers. Most of the members of the community attended the brief religious service. Then the slide projector was brought out and attached to the generator in the Land-Rover by means of the electrical cord. After that a series of color slides depicting the seven days of creation was shown, accompanied by a running commentary in the Koho language. It was a delightful presentation and the audience was obviously well pleased. These tribespeople could neither read nor write, but they understood these pictures because of previous exposure to such visual aids, and their knowledge of Bible stories, prayers and hymns would put many a Sunday School class to shame.

There were several young men whose minds were obviously not on the evening's Bible story and they repeatedly interrupted the leader with questions. He would laugh and he finally explained to us that they were anxious to be off on the evening's hunting expedition. At about nine o'clock the program was over and most of the villagers returned to their homes. Those who were visiting from surrounding areas found places to spend the night, though a few chose to file back through the forest to nearby homes, their burning torches lighting their way. And at last it was time for the safari.

When I had learned that our excursion would include a nighttime hunt, I promised myself, half in jest, to come back with a tiger skin. So I joined the group in the cab of the Land-Rover, while the young men of the village, armed with the guns provided by my host, sat on the roof of the car. With his bright searchlights they peered into the darkness as we drove slowly along the quiet deserted roads, looking for shining eyes that would betray the presence of the animals. Sambar deer, wild buffalo, wild pig, and civet cats abound in the area. Suddenly the stillness of the night was shattered by the sound of rifles from over our heads. The car stopped. A quick foray into the jungle proved that the target, whatever it might have been, had been missed. We continued on our way but, much to our disappointment, our night's only prize was one poor bedraggled rabbit.

After the morning church service, which was held in the still unfinished building, we broke camp and returned to Dalat. That evening, sitting about the fireplace, our host regaled us with stories of previous, more successful, safaris, perhaps hoping to compensate us for our disappointment, as well as reinstate himself in our minds as the number one game hunter of Vietnam. I, for one, believed him, for the tiger skin on which I sat was testimony to his skill.

A successful hunting expedition was, I told myself, probably too much to expect from my last trip to Dalat before returning to the States.

21

WHEN I RETURNED from Dalat the hospital's new wing was almost completed, but the most disruptive and noisiest work still remained to be done. While the workmen hammered and sawed, we attempted to go about our business. But the din of construction on top of the usual din of hundreds of clinic patients did not help our efficiency or concentration.

One blustery Saturday morning at the beginning of October when Dr. Yoder and I were in the midst of a heavy surgery schedule, a young woman carrying a baby was literally blown through the Chan-Y-Vien door into the reception room. With her was Kim Hoa smiling happily. The child, about a year old, with its large dark eyes and blond hair, had clearly been fathered by an American soldier.

I invited them to sit down in the doctor's office. The little girl sat quietly on her mother's lap while Kim Hoa explained that the woman was a friend of hers whose baby she had talked about to the Yoders some time before.

I flew to call Dr. Yoder, who was visiting patients in the ward. As soon as he joined the two young women, I ran to the house to tell Phyllis the exciting news, and she immediately went to the hospital to join her husband.

We later learned the circumstances that brought this young mother and her child to see the Yoders. She had learned from Kim Hoa that the Yoders wished to adopt a daughter but so far had been unsuccessful. Her family was wealthy, so it was not because of the possibility of remuneration that she had come. Although many mothers of half-foreign children had been selling their babies for large sums, this mother wanted neither money nor favors in return for her child. Because of the attractiveness of the baby she had had many offers of adoption, but until this time had refused to be parted from her daughter. Now, however, she was about to marry a Vietnamese officer. The marriage could not take place until another home was found for this child who, looking so different from the other children the woman would have, might be a source of embarrassment for the new family. She loved her baby dearly but realized that a home with an American family would be the best solution.

At the time, the child was flushed, running a high temperature and coughing. Dr. Yoder diagnosed pneumonia and, after a thorough examination, found that in all other respects she was a normal, healthy little girl. Then the mother and baby, Kim Hoa, and the Yoders went to the bungalow where they could continue their discussion of the child's future in private and without the coming and going of curious patients and bystanders.

Perhaps because of her illness, the baby was restless and clung to her mother, looking about with her beautiful eyes.

For a moment she allowed Phyllis to hold her, but then got restless again and was soon quieted only in the arms of her mother.

Suddenly the mother announced that she had decided to give them the baby right then, after only this brief conversation. She told the Yoders she believed they would love and protect her and that she would always be happy as their daughter.

The Yoders, startled that the mother could have made such a decision so quickly and with such finality, suggested that she take the baby home and weigh her decision first. But she insisted that she had considered every aspect of the matter and was satisfied that she was doing the right thing. She asked them to go with her immediately to the Province Chief's office, so that she could sign the necessary papers.

There was, tragically, a large black market in unwanted babies going on at the time. Many Vietnamese were buying children, promising the mothers to bring them up well, and actually using them as servants in their homes. To halt these practices the government had recently promulgated a new series of laws governing adoptions. The parent giving up the child had to sign a document relinquishing all claims to it. The adopting parents both had to be over thirty, married ten years with no children, and, of course, had to offer proof of an adequate income. Since Phyllis was in her late twenties and the Yoders had been married only six years, they would have to get special dispensation to make any adoption possible. But they knew that there was always a way to get around a law in Vietnam.

The Longacres were staying with us that weekend. Paul Longacre accompanied Phyllis and the mother to get the papers started on their long journey from the Provincial Government offices. Dr. Yoder joined me at the hospital and

Doris Longacre was left to tend the now fretful baby. The Yoders had long ago chosen a name—Susan—for the little girl they hoped to find, and now Susan was here.

The red tape of adoption went on through months of agonizing waiting. It involved several trips to Saigon to file new forms as old ones became dated and much effort on the part of various friends and government officials. The Longacres' interpreter, Ninh, who had worked for the Lichtis also, was ultimately credited with accomplishing the job. Ninh had friends in Saigon who, somehow, were always able to put the Yoders' papers on the very top of the right pile. One of the last necessary papers, waiving certain of the government regulations, had to be signed by Premier Khanh himself. We heard later that Khanh's attention had been called to the need for signing the document by a friend of Ninh's while he was attending a state funeral; and that it was one of the last papers to receive his signature before he was deposed in February of 1965. Even after that it took several more months before the adoption was finalized, and it wasn't until shortly before they were to leave the following July that the Yoders gratefully had in their possession the sheaf of forms declaring that Susan was officially and irrevocably Susan Yoder.

The grandparents who had never seen her sent all kinds of things for Suzy to wear and play with. She slept in the crib that had been left behind by Dr. Dick. And after only a few weeks she ate while sitting in a high chair. It was made by one of our night workers from a picture in a magazine advertisement which I had shown him. It was quite, quite high— much larger than the one it was patterned after, since there was no way for the amateur carpenter to judge the size of the one in the advertisement—but it was very sturdy and the baby looked adorable in it.

The presence of a child in the bungalow brought about a delightful change for all of us. Although the adjustment was difficult for Susan, who was old enough to miss the mother she had known, Phyllis' and the doctor's love and patience eventually overcame her early insecurity. Although she had never before eaten many of the foods now given her, she took the changes in her diet as a matter of course, but she made her likes and dislikes known. Susan was adamant in her refusal of milk and, surprisingly, sweets.

Phyllis now devoted herself almost exclusively to caring for her new daughter. Anh Ba was especially privileged, because Susan at once decided she loved him. Anh Ba would often be able to reverse an otherwise unhappy moment for both Susan and Phyllis by his timely arrival on the scene. He adored the baby and they spent many happy hours together, she on a mat in the kitchen while he cooked and baked for our meals, talking to her in Vietnamese and in the few words of English he knew. Most frequently the English word was "No," but it was always said gently. When Susan learned to walk, her first stroll all by herself was from our home to Anh Ba's small house near by. Here Susan joined his wife and four children as naturally and happily as if they were her own family.

Missy, our watchdog, somehow knew that Susan was very special and though she never allowed the baby to touch her she would always watch when Susan played in the yard or went for a walk. Missy allowed no stranger near Susan, as several people can testify, having had their trousers slashed by her teeth when they ignored her presence.

Christmas that year was for Susan and was the happiest anyone of us had had in a long time. Gifts from friends and relatives were heaped around the base of our sparkling aluminum Christmas tree. Susan did all the right things, opening presents, trying out toys, putting on and taking off hats and clothes—performing all the delightful tricks a fourteen-month-old girl has special knowledge of.

Soon afterward I learned that my father would once more be coming to Nhatrang to see me during his tour of leprosariums in Southeast Asia. I looked forward to being able to show him our expanding facilities. I knew he would appreciate the changes that had taken place since his first visit nearly three years ago, just after my arrival.

I had been thinking about the future, knowing that my term of service in Vietnam would soon be over and that I must plan for what was to follow. But the thought of leaving was a disturbing one. And when the M.C.C. notified me that they would not have a nurse to replace me by February, when my original contract would end, I was not too sorry. I had written them that I would like to enter a second term of service with them. I wanted to try a change of country, culture and religion, possibly in an Arab land, and they wrote that I might be able to serve in Algeria. But in the meantime my contract was extended first to April, and later to July. I was happy to know that the Yoders would be leaving at about the same time, for by now because of all we had shared and experienced together it would have been difficult to adjust to working with someone new. Dr. Yoder's replacement was to arrive in April when Dr. Yoder would still be on hand to offer guidance.

Because of Susan the Yoders were looking forward to going home that summer. Both sets of grandparents, as well as hosts of friends, were anxious to see their new daughter.

Dad came at the end of January, detouring from his itinerary for a quick trip to the Chan-Y-Vien. This time, unfortunately, there could be no trip to the leprosarium at Ban-methuot. Following the kidnapping there, now more than two years ago, the remaining American missionary staff had had to leave the grounds and move into town, leaving the leprosarium in the care of only the native Rhadde staff, which they had trained. From headquarters established in the city of Banmethuot the Americans continued to supply drugs and give guidance and training to the Rhadde work-ers. They were also able to conduct mobile clinics in nearby villages, bringing medicines to known patients and diagnos-ing and treating new cases. Periodically the villages where they held clinic in the daytime would be occupied after dark by the Vietcong, but still their health-preserving work con-tinued. And the Rhadde staff at the leprosarium proved apt and faithful, for there, too, the work continued. Even surgi-cal procedures, we heard, were being done by one of the Rhadde men. This tribesman had been trained over a period of several years by Dr. Vietti and the other physicians. As for the three kidnapped Americans, they have not yet been heard from, except indirectly. The International Red Cross at one time received word from their captors that they were well and could receive packages and letters. Food, clothing, and mail were sent, but no reply was ever received.

My father's visit to Nhatrang was a pleasant one. In spite of the increasingly alarming news about Vietnam in the American press, he was not overly concerned for my safety. His own previous experiences in a strife-torn country gave him an understanding of such situations. He remembered that he had had comparative safety and freedom to work in even though he had been surrounded by a war in Assam in the 1940's. And so our conversation that day dealt more with news of home and family and with my work.

But unpredictable events continued to keep the political

202

situation an ever-present reality. While Dad was there the Buddhists staged another demonstration, this time in Nhatrang. Buddhist monks fasted in the main square as a means of demanding that General Khanh, President of South Vietnam, agree to step from power. Some monks spoke over public microphones to the crowds that gathered, while others led orderly processions of quietly chanting and praying men and women through the city streets. I observed these activities on a trip to town and, standing aside to allow one procession to pass, I recognized several former patients in the crowd. They acknowledged me with faint smiles. The demonstrations were orderly, causing no real disruption, and after two days all was again calm. Elsewhere in the country demonstrations and rioting continued. Student leaders from Saigon came to Nhatrang hoping to stir up further activity, but they were essentially unsuccessful.

One afternoon while the student leaders were in Nhatrang, a large party of them went for a swim in the ocean. Two students, a boy and a girl, swam out farther than the others and became exhausted. When the girl panicked, the boy tried to help her. When the rest of the group saw him floundering they began to shout for help. Two American G.I.s swimming near by quickly went to their aid with the help of a Vietnamese fishing boat. They reached the victims and pulled them into the boat. But when they tried to revive the two, only the girl responded. One of the G.I.s hastened over to the Province Hospital and returned with the U.S. O.M. surgeon and special equipment. By the time both students were removed to the Province Hospital, it was obvious that the girl would survive, but the boy was beyond recall.

Soon an angry crowd of young people was milling about the compound of the Province Hospital, demanding to talk with the doctor and the Americans and also to be allowed to see the girl. They were angry that it was the girl who had been saved, accusing the Americans of not having tried hard enough to save the boy. The U.S.O.M. doctor calmly spoke to them, explaining that everything possible had been done. As for the girl, the doctor explained that she needed rest, which she surely would not have if they all insisted on visiting her. He suggested that they elect five or six of their number to act as representatives, and he gave them his word that this delegation would be admitted to her bedside. Soon afterward the crowd dispersed. Later six of them came back to visit the girl and were admitted as the doctor promised.

Two days later an elaborate Buddhist funeral was staged for the boy, attended by most of the students in Nhatrang and many from Saigon. Friends and family members from Saigon came as well, swelling the ranks of the enormous, noisier-than-usual procession that followed the hearse. In a *xich-lo* at the head of the line, weeping, could be seen the still exhausted girl whose life had been saved. Everyone was relieved when this incident finally ended.

The day Dad left Vietnam, General Khanh was deposed and a civilian government headed by Pham Huy Quat took control. A short while after that, capitalizing on the government's political crisis, Vietcong guerrillas attacked the U.S. Army installation at Pleiku. Several American servicemen were killed, more wounded.

Following a similar attack on the base at Quinhon some time later, Washington retaliated by ordering U.S. bombers to blast various targets in North Vietnam. There were rumors that an announcement of the deployment of U.S. Marines and Army combat units to South Vietnam would come momentarily.

All dependents of U.S. servicemen and government employees residing in South Vietnam were ordered to leave the country within 24 or 48 hours. The only exceptions were single American women working at essential jobs and, of course, personnel not in the employ of the U.S. government. Since this category included us, we were not under obligation to leave. The Army, however, kindly offered to evacuate us all to Saigon. When we stated our desire and intention to remain, we were told that it would be at our own risk, and that the Army could not consider itself responsible for our safety in the event of further danger. Their offer to evacuate us as far as Saigon would still be good should the future warrant it.

Within a week another military coup in the continuing game of "capture the flag" took place. Pham Huy Quat was ousted. General Khanh attempted to regain the premiership. And life went on.

22

IN THE SPRING when the monsoon season should have been past, a series of terrible storms lashed our area as well as other parts of Vietnam. Two stretches of the road at the foot of the lane leading from the hospital were washed away by monstrous waves, leaving us virtually isolated. Our only access to the main paved road was now the road through the orphanage grounds, so every trip to town took us through the gates of that institution. As these gates were kept locked, small boys, part of the orphanage's family, were made responsible for opening and locking the gates after traffic had passed. One of the most cheerful, quick and appealing of these gatekeepers was Ninh, a little nine-year-old boy, one of only five tribal children at the orphanage (the rest being Vietnamese or French-Vietnamese).

Ninh had never known his father. His mother was killed during a government raid on her village, which was occupied

206

by rebel forces. His two older brothers had already left the village of their parents and both were soldiers in the Vietnamese Army. After the raid, Ninh was found by an U.S. Army major and taken to live at a camp near Pleiku. Ninh spoke of a happy life there, where he had obviously made himself the company pet with his quick mind, sparkling eyes, and eager intelligence. He learned to speak his own brand of English, colorfully spiced with the usual G.I. slang, which sounded so much more expressive coming from this small bundle of energy. The major, having become deeply attached to the boy, requested permission from Ninh's older brothers to adopt him. They decided they could not allow him to be taken away permanently. And so, when the major's tour came to an end, Ninh once more had to adjust to another way of life—this time the Vietnamese life as it was lived in the Protestant orphanage near the Chan-Y-Vien.

He had never learned Vietnamese, having spoken the tribal language for most of his years and English for the last two. When he arrived at the orphanage he still could not speak Vietnamese and he had forgotten much of his native tribal tongue while living with the Americans. So he would come to visit us at the hospital to practice his English and to be around some Americans while he was learning Vietnamese.

Additional torrential rains inland in the wake of the tidal storms had flooded several villages, whose luckless inhabitants had been forced to flee to higher ground. Only nine miles from the hospital was a town that was badly flood damaged and during the inhabitants' absence it was taken over by the Vietcong. This tactic was not infrequent with the Vietcong. As soon as they learned that a village had been abandoned they moved in, even before the waters subsided. When the owners returned, they could retrieve their property only after making a pledge of loyalty, usually in the tangible form of a tax or donation.

This was one of the few times the Vietcong became entrenched so close to the hospital. Our work, however, continued, affected only to the extent that patients living in this nearby area now found it difficult to get to us because of Vietcong control of traffic in and out of the village. At least one patient from that village, an old woman who had diabetes, had been threatened when she tried to come to the hospital for medication.

During three particularly busy days of one week that last spring, we treated two cases of near-fatal snake bite, delivered two babies, did five eye surgery procedures and three other minor surgery cases, treated one case of tetanus, vainly attempted to revive a little girl brought to us after drowning, saw over seven hundred patients in clinic, made two emergency trips to the Province Hospital, and got a total of no more than nine hours' sleep.

Once things calmed down at the hospital we began hearing more and more about the increased activities of the Vietcong in our own area and throughout all of South Vietnam. Secretary of Defense Robert S. McNamara was then touring Southeast Asia and most of the news reports we received over the radio dealt with his trip and his speeches. His most recent talk, delivered in Manila, assured his audience that all U.S. military personnel would be withdrawn from South Vietnam before the end of 1965. He inferred that the Vietcong were being driven back and would soon surrender, thus bringing the war to a victorious conclusion.

It seemed impossible that the Secretary of Defense didn't know what we, with our limited access to information, felt we knew only too well. The Vietcong seemed stronger than they had ever been and held at least 50 per cent of South

Vietnamese territory. Furthermore, more and more men and materiel were arriving in Vietnam daily. In Nhatrang alone, the buildup of troops and military equipment was progressing at a frightening pace. This kind of talk was to reassure the American public. But for us it served only to increase our concern over the seeming disparity between fact and propaganda. Why was the American public not being allowed to know the truth of the situation in Vietnam?

Our information about what was occurring in the capital was spotty but I had a chance to find out more a short time later. Dr. Yoder gave me what was described, with tongue in cheek, as a three-day pass to Saigon. It would combine business and pleasure. The business was to purchase medicine. The pleasure part was the relaxation of staying with the Longacres in their pretty two-storied French villa.

During the flight down I was able to see a vast new installation being built by the United States. Cam Ranh Bay, a 75-mile stretch of deep water which lay behind a long, uninhabited peninsula that began 31 miles below Nhatrang, was being developed as a military staging area and to provide anchorage for American naval ships. From the plane I could see that it was well on its way to completion. Already the almost landlocked harbor was filled with a variety of ships including L.S.T.s and freighters. It was a sharp and conclusive contradiction of Secretary McNamara's pledge to withdraw American forces and, I thought, an ironic comment on a war which was already filled with too many other unhappy ironies.

When we arrived at the Saigon-Tansonnhut Airport I saw further evidence of American commitment to the war. Ostensibly Tansonnhut was operated by the Vietnamese; but there were many more uniformed American personnel. In 1962 the airport had had only one jet runway; now there were several. There were more fighter planes than I could begin to count, a new control tower, radar equipment, and at the edge of the field barbed wire fences heavily patrolled by armed soldiers. At strategic points there were anti-aircraft guns and mobile weapon carriers mounted with machine guns. Just two years before, Tansonnhut was still a small and simple field designed solely to handle commercial traffic. Now it was an armed military field.

Saigon, of course, had also grown into an armed camp. But the new population of American military personnel did not detract from the gaiety of a city that had more in common with sophisticated European capitals than with the usual Asiatic towns. In fact, the G.I.s added to the frantic pace.

After I arrived at the Longacres', we received an invitation to dinner from one of their Vietnamese friends. We left the house in an M.C.C.-owned Ford Falcon, a luxurious vehicle in comparison with our Volkswagen pickup and, after meeting companions who were driving their own newly purchased foreign car, we plunged into a night on the town that was quite unlike anything I had seen since the last time I was in New York.

I couldn't remember when I had given myself so fully to having a good time. Wherever we went that evening, people were laughing, dancing, and enjoying the pleasures of a gay city. The mood was infectious and it was hard to remember that the country was at war. Marquees and billboards advertised entertainers who performed popular American songs. Even hillbilly music could be heard. Beautiful Vietnamese girls in lovely and often very expensive *ao dais* walked along the streets with their Vietnamese or American escorts, looking into shop windows full of all kinds of merchandise— stereo sets and radios, cosmetics and clothes, mostly imported from Europe or the United States. Restaurants featured a variety of cuisines—Chinese, Vietnamese, French and American—and attracted as many nationalities. There was heavy traffic along all the main streets, and from the number of shining new vehicles one could scarcely credit the reports of waiting lists of several years for new cars.

When I boarded the plane for Nhatrang and flew once again over the city called the Paris of the East, I was reminded of how alien to the rest of Vietnam Saigon seemed to be, how removed the center of the city was from the realities lying outside of its limits. And yet this was the seat of the government, the pulse, the capital of the country.

The Chan-Y-Vien's new wing was ready at last. Even before the beds and other furnishings were in place we had put it to use for some patients, who just placed their mats right on the floor. On the day our big drug order finally arrived the Blue Goose was reactivated to bring the shipment up from the waterfront. Attracted by the large crates and general hubbub, neighbors gathered to get in on the activity. We soon realized that many of them wanted to acquire the empty wooden packing cases, and to avoid chaos we instituted a game somewhat resembling the drawing for door prizes at a ladies' luncheon. Everyone joined in and the winners were particularly delighted with their prizes.

We were now able to accommodate as many as 48 patients in our new and old wards. One evening just as we were finishing our final rounds of the wards, one of the children, a seven-year-old boy with a severe chronic heart ailment, quietly died. His mother had been watching over him and, when she realized what had happened, immediately began to gather her few belongings and make preparations to leave. I gently reminded her that it was well past the curfew hour, too late to hire public transportation to take her and her boy home. She looked at me blankly, seemingly unable to comprehend anything but the fact of her child's death. Knowing how important it is for these people to be at home when death occurs, or as soon as possible afterward, I asked where she lived. I would try to get her home. She told me the name of her village, a small one about nine miles to the west.

I told Anh Tin that I was going to take the mother and boy home. He replied that the village lay in Vietcong-controlled territory and that it would be impossible for me to get through. When the mother was told this, she said she needed transportation only to the home of a brother who lived within safe territory, on the other side of Nhatrang, supposedly under the jurisdiction of the city. From there on, she explained, she could easily get help from members of her family.

After a long conversation with the woman, Anh Tin told me it might be possible to get her to her brother's house. Then he announced that he would accompany me. He was dressed in his white trousers and shirt and I was in uniform. With the woman's strong reassurance that she knew the area and people where we were going, both Anh Tin and I felt relatively secure. But I did get a little shaken when Anh Tin said, "Be prepared to drive off quickly if you hear any shooting."

Our trip into Nhatrang followed the very familiar road and our minds dwelt not on it where we knew we never had anything to fear, but on the road that we would take out of the city into the dark, quiet countryside of rice fields and tiny gardens, children and flowers, so well known and familiar during the day and in the sunlight, but now so deserted and somehow sinister because of our imaginations in the dark.

212

We passed the checkpoint on the city's western limits, stopping to identify ourselves and our purpose for leaving the city. At first the guard seemed startled at our venturing on such a journey after curfew. But when Ahn Tin explained the circumstances he allowed us to pass, warning us to go no further than a specific bridge which he described. If we crossed this bridge, we would be outside of the safe territory. As we pulled away from the checkpoint, Anh Tin told me that the guard was related to a child who had been a patient at the Chan-Y-Vien the previous year and was acquainted with the work of the hospital. Perhaps for this reason he allowed us to pass without much ado.

On we sped along the good paved road, the headlights showing nothing but the empty road ahead. Anh Tin and I talked quietly while the woman sat huddled over her child in the back of the Volkswagen, now and again directing us through the open window between the cab and the back of the truck.

Just before we approached the bridge, the woman instructed me to slow down and stop. The truck came to a halt. All was quiet except for the shrill call of the crickets. I turned off all but the parking lights of the car and, as I did so, the woman climbed down and disappeared from view. My eyes had not yet accustomed themselves to the blackness of the unlit night and I could not see where she had gone. In the silence I could hear my heart pounding. I wondered if Anh Tin, too, was afraid. But I did not dare to break the silence.

A small beam of light flashed. I could make out a kerosene lamp and the woman approaching a small house. We heard her calling softly at the gate to identify herself and we saw a man, presumably her brother, unlock the gate and join her. They walked back to us. The man quietly greeted me and then put his hand on the child's head. "Your son is dead," he murmured. "Yes, brother," she sobbed. "He was too sick too long for the doctor to save him."

Out of nowhere came two black-clad figures carrying a makeshift stretcher on which they gently laid the boy's body. Then they carried it off into the all-encompassing night. After gathering her few bundles with the help of her brother she thanked me for what we had done. Then she was gone.

I had remained in the truck all the while, afraid that even the small beam of light shining on my white uniform would attract too much attention. The brother was saying, "Go quickly now. Do not remain here longer—and thank you for caring for my sister's son."

I was only too happy to comply with his wishes and reached out to turn on the ignition. Out of the darkness came a sharply spoken "Stop." My heart stopped beating and my blood froze.

On the bridge in front of us stood three men in black. The parking lights glinted on the guns in their hands. Their command had cracked through the quiet night like a shot. But the dead boy's uncle moved immediately to them. Anxiously I strained to hear his words. He explained our mission and I caught my breath.

They lowered their guns. When he had finished, the three figures silently walked about inspecting the Volkswagen. Anh Tin and I sat still, looking straight ahead.

Then one of them nodded. We were dismissed. I said the traditional words of farewell to a man, "Chao ong," and gratefully started the motor, turned the truck about and headed back to Nhatrang.

We drove in silence for several miles. Then Anh Tin asked if I knew that they had been village defense militiamen, responsible for guarding the bridge and its environs. So they had not been Vietcong after all. My fears, fortunately, had been for nothing. He then asked me if I had been afraid. When I admitted that I had been, he admitted that he had been too. He had only realized at the end that they were not rebel soldiers. "All I could think was who would care for my wife and three children if those men were Vietcong and decided to kidnap or shoot us," he said.

We passed the checkpoint, once again stopping to identify ourselves and allow the truck to be given a perfunctory inspection. We told the guard that all had gone well. His parting remark was, "I hope the rest of this night passes as quietly and uneventfully as that which has already passed." It was our wish for him too, as we drove off.

DATE DUE